Praise for Ea

D0390070

"This inspired and well-researched book explains the perils we face by being disconnected from the power and energy of the Earth and its boundless storehouse of free electrons. Could much of the disease, chronic inflammation, poor sleep, and more be the result of this? A brilliant hypothesis well-grounded in science."
—NICHOLAS PERRICONE, M.D.,
AUTHOR OF *AGELESS FACE, AGELESS MIND*

"Earthing ranks right up there with the discovery of penicillin. This book is probably the most important health read of the twenty-first century."
—ANN LOUISE GITTLEMAN, PH.D., C.N.S.,
AUTHOR OF *THE FAT FLUSH PLAN*

TOP 10 SPA AND WELLNESS TRENDS FOR 2013
"As modern-day humans become more cut off from nature, Earthing specifically refers to the movement promoting direct contact with the earth's electron-rich surface . . . to help combat 'nature deficit disorder.'"
—SpaFinder Wellness 10th Annual Forecast based on surveys of global spa and wellness businesses, travel agents, and consumers

Earthing
The most important health discovery ever!

Clinton Ober
Stephen T. Sinatra, M.D.
Martin Zucker

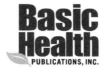
Basic Health
PUBLICATIONS, INC.

The information contained in this book is based upon the research and personal and professional experiences of the authors. It is not intended as a substitute for consulting with your physician or other healthcare provider. Any attempt to diagnose and treat an illness should only be done under the direction of a healthcare professional.

The publisher does not advocate the use of any particular healthcare protocol but believes the information in this book should be available to the public. The publisher and authors are not responsible for any adverse effects or consequences resulting from the use of the ideas or procedures discussed in this book. Should the reader have any questions, the authors and the publisher strongly suggest consulting a professional healthcare advisor.

Basic Health Publications, Inc.
28812 Top of the World Drive
Laguna Beach, CA 92651
949-715-7327 • www.basichealthpub.com

Library of Congress Cataloging-in-Publication Data

Ober, Clinton
 Earthing : the most important health discovery ever! / by Clinton
Ober, Stephen T. Sinatra, and Martin Zucker.
   p. cm.
 Includes bibliographical references and index.
 ISBN 978-1-59120-374-2
 1. Electromagnetism in medicine. 2. Electromagnetism—Physiological
effect. I. Sinatra, Stephen T. II. Zucker, Martin III. Title.
  RZ422.O24   2014
  612.01442—dc22
                                                    2009048101

Editor: Cheryl Hirsch
Typesetting/Book design: Gary A. Rosenberg
Cover design: Clinton Ober and The Design Partnership
Illustrations: W. Peter Pauley Jr., The Design Partnership, Colorado Springs, CO

Printed in the United States of America

10   9   8   7   6   5   4

Contents

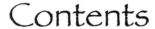

PART FOUR:
The Earthing Chronicles

Appendices

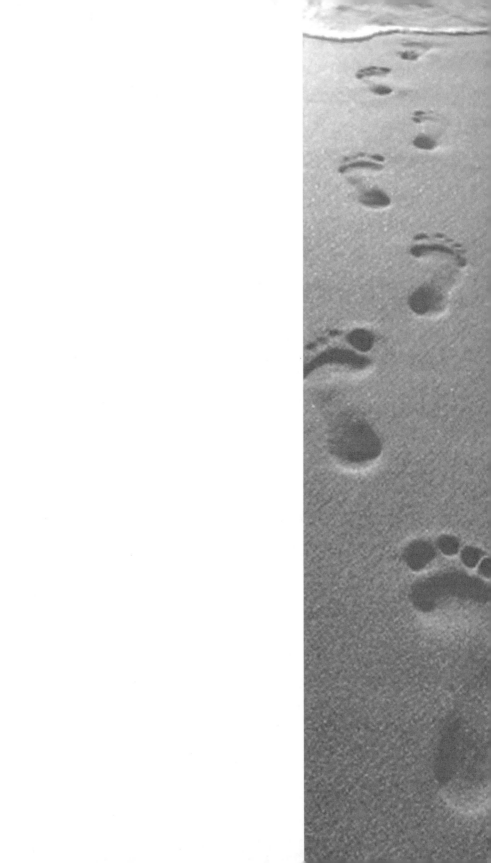

Foreword

By James L. Oschman, Ph.D.
Author of *Energy Medicine: The Scientific Basis* and
Energy Medicine in Therapeutics and Human Performance

This book unfolds an amazing story of discovery, a process that you, the reader, will soon experience for yourself as you read through the pages ahead.

It is a rare and humbling experience for a scientist to have the opportunity to explore new ground—and this story is all about ground—and participate in research that quickly infuses better health and more happiness into people's lives. It has been an exciting and challenging process for me. I was forced to ask questions that had never been asked before. The answers have ranged from fascinating to astounding, and they have shed light on some of the most important unsolved problems in physiology and medicine.

Among the many surprising revelations this book holds is an obvious, fundamental, and yet overlooked answer to the question of inflammation —recognized as the central health issue of our time—that surely will lay the foundation for many academic investigations and doctoral projects well into the future. To get an idea of the impact of inflammation on health, refer to Figure 1 on the next page. It tracks the dramatic proliferation of scientific studies on inflammation—now approaching 30,000 a year!—for nearly a half-century. Inflammation is thus being revealed as a critical link between our lifestyle and the soaring global increase of chronic diseases— the biggest health problems both in terms of cost and human suffering.

These revelations place the book you are about to read at the center of the most significant health issue in our modern age.

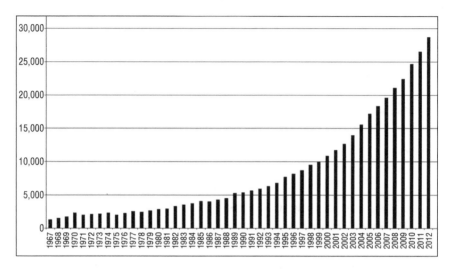

Figure 1. Year-by-year increase of published peer-reviewed studies on inflammation, 1967–2012. Source: Pub Med (National Library of Medicine database), as of January 2013.

I say that without equivocation, as an experienced academic cell biologist and biophysicist who has published dozens of articles in some of the world's leading scientific journals. The research in this book puts forward, and from a completely unexpected direction, a powerful explanation for the proliferation of inflammation and, most important, what we can do about it.

As you read this book, you will quickly learn some profound and life-impacting facts you never knew before about our relationship with the planet we live on. You'll learn, for instance, how electrons play a central role in this relationship. The role of electrons in biology and health has long been my favorite subject. Of special importance in my explorations of the electronic aspects of life was an association during the 1980s with the leading research group studying this subject, consisting of Nobel Laureate Albert Szent-Györgyi and colleagues from around the world at the Marine Biological Laboratory in Woods Hole, Massachusetts. A number of these great inquiring minds were electronic engineers and materials scientists recruited to study a field he created and named *electronic biology*.

Dr. Szent-Györgyi was considered one of the leading scientists of the twentieth century, and his research and writings have been a continuing source of inspiration and insight. I have published a series of articles and two books on the ways electrons can move about within the human body and the ways various therapeutic methods influence electron motions. The research summarized in this book adds a whole new dimension to our understandings of electronic biology.

The book traces the discoveries of Clinton Ober, a pioneer in the cable TV industry, who uncovered real health benefits from "Earthing," his term for being barefoot outside or in bare-skin contact with special conductive sheets and mats indoors that are connected to the ground. Many people describe a significant sense of well-being as a result of Earthing.

The stories and the research in the book reveal the background, dynamics, and implications of this feel-good sensation, a real experience indicative of something profoundly important that most of us have been missing in our lives. This missing link is so profound in fact that it seems to do away with or dramatically improve so many health challenges common in this day and age: insomnia, the chronic pain of multiple diseases and injuries, exhaustion, stress, anxiety, and premature aging. Even the most superbly conditioned individuals—elite athletes—recover much faster from their exertions and injuries.

I was quickly and enthusiastically drawn into this research when I saw how many people experienced a wide variety of health and recovery benefits from simply connecting their bodies to the Earth. When my massage therapist began using Earthing with her clients, she achieved so many successes that physicians in the area began sending her their most difficult cases to treat. My challenge was to help determine precisely how Earthing produces such effects and to explain it as accurately as possible in the language of science.

Other researchers, from as far apart as California and Eastern Europe, have joined in this fascinating project. Our explorations have uncovered what is perhaps the most simple and natural remedy against proliferating, painful, and often deadly conditions, including the diseases of aging, created by various kinds of inflammation. As you will read further on, our hypothesis for how this remedy works is unlike any you have ever heard. In all its ramifications, we think it represents a new healing paradigm.

In short, Earthing restores and maintains the human body's most natural electrical state, which in turn promotes optimum health and functionality in daily life. The primordial natural energy emanating from the Earth is the ultimate anti-inflammatory and the ultimate antiaging medicine.

For more than fifteen years, Clint Ober has tirelessly pursued a mission to awaken a skeptical world to a simple and forgotten fact: that the Earth beneath our feet contains great healing energy and that connecting ourselves to this energy is immediately beneficial as well as intuitively and remarkably simple.

As with any new discovery, Clint had to endure skepticism and derision from "experts," some of whom regarded him as crazy. But he persisted and has now gathered significant scientific evidence for his out-of-the-box idea. Moreover, many thousands of people who have applied the concept of Earthing in their lives feel, look, and sleep better, and they have less pain.

As we explored absolutely new avenues of research in order to validate the concept of Earthing and determine how it affects the human body, Clint turned out to be a rock solid and dedicated guide to those of us with Ph.D.s after our names. Clint often refers to his lack of education as a scientist, but what he has accomplished shows that determined and inspired individuals can accomplish an enormous amount by teaching themselves what they need to know. I have been continually astonished by his precise and accurate insights that go beyond the conclusions a logical scientific mind would usually develop. I feel that I have been privileged to work with a genuine discoverer and pioneer whose interest in helping others exceeds any personal interest by far.

Steve Sinatra, a Connecticut cardiologist who specializes in integrative medicine and has an interest in electromedicine, met Clint in 2001 and saw great promise for Earthing in his own field of cardiology, as well as medicine in general. Steve encouraged Clint to stick with it and pursue research, particularly the connection with inflammation, which had been found to be the probable cause of heart disease.

In 2010, Clint, Steve, and veteran health-writer Martin Zucker teamed up to write the fascinating Earthing story as a book. Since its publication, the book has been translated into more than a dozen languages. This second edition contains additional research and evidence of the Earth's potent healing properties.

To break new ground means to do something different from anything done before. If ever the term *groundbreaking* applies to a book, it certainly does here, literally and figuratively. This book is about the ground beneath our feet, and the revelation of a vital electrical continuum between the Earth and the living organisms that dwell upon it.

Walk, stand, and sit barefoot on the ground for a half hour or so. If you have PMS or arthritic pain or a backache or indigestion or jet lag or are just feeling fatigued, go outside (weather permitting, of course) with your bare feet placed directly on the Earth.

At the end of that time you will feel better. And as you feel better, a lightbulb will go off in your head. You will realize that although you live on the surface of the Earth your lifestyle has separated you from the limitless healing energy that, unknown to you, the surface beneath your feet holds. It's there, and always there, and yours for the taking.

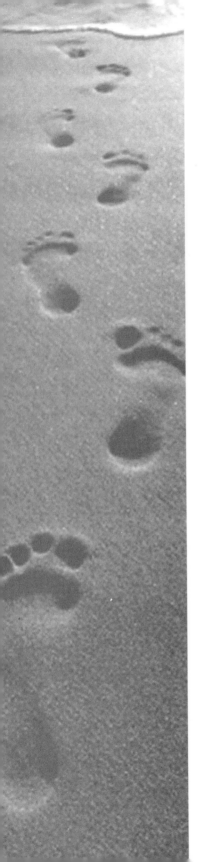

PART ONE

Why We Are Increasingly Unhealthy– The Missing Link

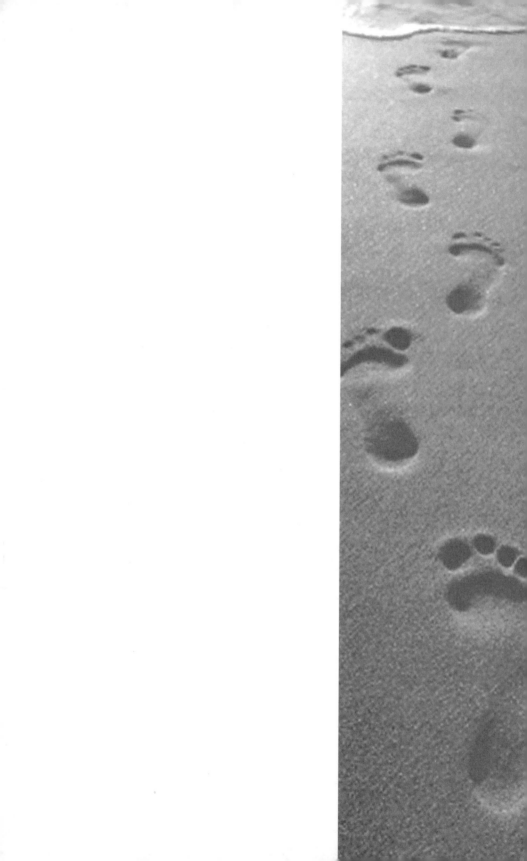

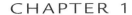

CHAPTER 1

The Miracle of Mother Earth

In all things of Nature there is something of the marvelous.
—ARISTOTLE

The Earth beneath our feet provides sustenance in the form of food and water. It provides a surface to sit, stand, walk, run, swim, climb, play, and build on. And, it also provides something very surprising and marvelous, something you likely never, ever thought about.

Healing power.

Marvelous healing power.

In the book you are about to read, you will learn about this eternal healing power, the astonishing magnitude of which was discovered through the curiosity and persistence of a few individuals.

If possible, sit with your bare feet directly on the Earth—grass, gravel, dirt, sand, or concrete—while you read. If you do, you will simultaneously make your own personal discovery and experience what you are reading about. You will feel a positive shift within you as your body becomes infused with the natural healing power of the Earth.

In this book you will also read about people from all over the world who connect to this unlikely power source with remarkable results. People such as these:

- A former attorney for a Fortune 500 company who experienced a dramatic remission from lupus, a devastating autoimmune disorder.

- An Australian doctor who restores feeling to the numb feet of patients suffering from diabetic neuropathy.

- A paraplegic in Alaska who was unable to move his feet for twenty-five years after an accident and is able now not only to move his feet but also to begin taking a few steps.

- And others suffering from common disorders who have gotten relief by reconnecting to Mother Earth.

We call the reconnection "Earthing" or "grounding."

WHAT IS EARTHING?

Earthing is both a timeless practice and a modern discovery. It simply means living in contact with the Earth's natural surface charge—being grounded—which naturally discharges and prevents chronic inflammation in the body. This effect has massive health implications because of the strong link between chronic inflammation and virtually all chronic disease, including the diseases of aging, and the aging process itself.

But don't we all live on the Earth? you may be thinking.

Yes, we live on Earth, but most of us don't touch the Earth anymore.

Throughout practically all of history, we humans have maintained a direct physical connection with the Earth—the skin of our bodies touching the skin of the Earth.

We walked barefoot and slept directly on the ground. We were at all times naturally charged with the healing energy of the Earth. Today, we mostly live and work insulated from the Earth. We wear nonconductive shoes with synthetic soles, walk on carpeted floors, and sleep in elevated beds. We do not live on the ground. We even live and work high off the ground, in high rises. We rarely go barefoot outside.

We're disconnected.

We're Earth-starved.

Consequently, our bodies have become chronically charged with inflammation, an unnatural development, and one that appears to represent an overlooked reason why immune dysfunction and inflammation-related health disorders have dramatically proliferated, ravaging adults and children alike. We've lost our electrical roots, the Earth's electrical ground that serves as our primordial anti-inflammatory protection.

Earthing offers a simple remedy for the disconnect. It's as easy as being barefoot outdoors or sleeping, working, and relaxing indoors on conductive systems designed for the house and office. Whether outdoors or indoors, you are reconnecting to the Earth's natural surface charge and restoring a natural electrical state in your physiology.

This book documents how reconnecting and grounding the body consistently produces these and other common benefits:

- Rapid reduction of inflammation.

- Rapid reduction or elimination of chronic pain.

- Dynamic blood flow improvement to better supply the cells and tissues of the body with vital oxygen and nutrition.

- Reduced stress.

- Increased energy.

- Improved sleep.

- Accelerated healing from injuries and surgery.

Earthing is among the most natural and safest things you can do to improve your health; something simple yet astoundingly profound. It is not a treatment but a hugely rewarding return-to-a-core aspect of Nature that we have abandoned. Earthing is a missing link in the health equation.

This book tells why and what to do about it.

The Most Important Health Discovery Ever? or The Most Important Health Discovery Ever!

In the first edition, the subtitle of our book ended with a question mark. For this, the second edition, we have chosen an exclamation point.

That's because we are even more convinced that reconnecting to the Earth represents a landmark health discovery, with great implications for our chronic disease-plagued society. About that we have no doubts and no question.

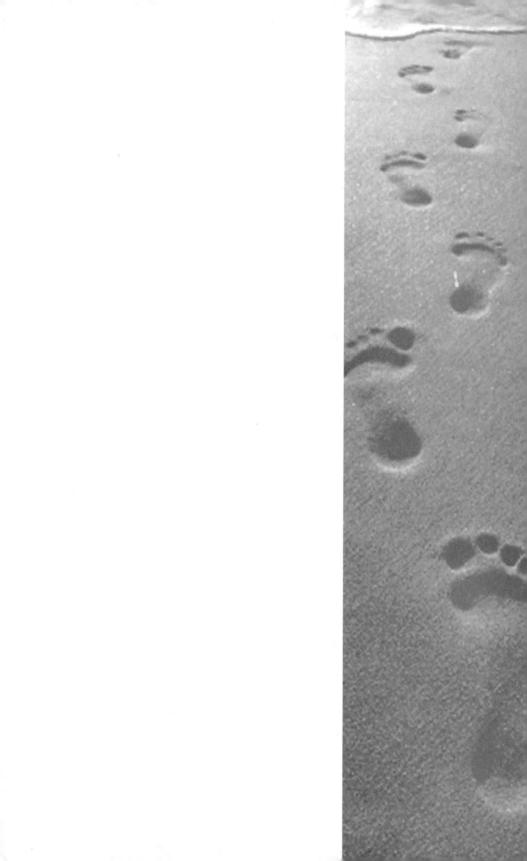

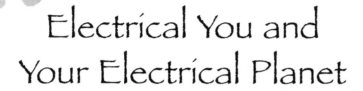

CHAPTER 2

Electrical You and Your Electrical Planet

Have you ever noticed a subtle tingling or sensation of warmth rising up from your feet during a barefoot stroll on a sandy beach or grassy field glistening with the morning dew?

Did you feel revitalized at the end of your walk?

If you did, you experienced the Earth energizing your body.

The fact is that we live on a planet alive with natural energies. Its surface teems with subtly pulsating frequencies, a phenomenon unknown to most people. Who regards the sand, grass, sidewalk, or dirt beneath their feet as an energy field?

But that indeed is what the ground is and always has been.

Put another way, your planet is a six sextillion (that's six followed by twenty-one zeroes) metric ton battery that is continually being replenished by solar radiation, lightning, and heat from its deep-down molten core. And just like a battery in a car that keeps the motor running and the wheels turning, so, too, do the rhythmic pulsations of natural energy flowing through and emanating from the surface of the Earth keep the biological machinery of global life running in rhythm and balance—for everything that lives on the land or in the sea.

People.

Animals.

Fish.

Plants.

Trees.

Bugs.

Bacteria.

Viruses.

Throughout history, humans have sat, stood, strolled, and slept on the ground without knowing that such simple contact transfers a natural electrical signal to the body.

Only recently has the knowledge and significance of this connection been explored and explained by scientific experts in geophysics, biophysics, electrical engineering, electrophysiology, and medicine. From them, we are learning that the Earth's electrical energy maintains the order of our own bodily frequencies just as a conductor controls the coherence and cadence of an orchestra. We all live and function electrically on an electrical planet. We are each of us a collection of dynamic electrical circuits in which trillions of cells constantly transmit and receive energy in the course of their programmed biochemical reactions. Think of them as microscopic electronic machines. The movement of nutrients and water into the cells is regulated by electric fields, and each type of cell has a frequency range in which it operates. Your heart, brain, nervous system, muscles, and immune system are prime examples of electrical subsystems operating within your bioelectrical body. The fact is, all of your movements, behaviors, and actions are energized by electricity.

OUR LOST ELECTRICAL ROOTS

Most people, even in this scientific age, are totally unaware of their bioelectrical nature. Practically no one has the slightest notion of an electrical or energetic connection between his or her body and the Earth. Nobody learns about it in school. So nobody knows that we have largely become disconnected and separated from the Earth. In developed societies, in particular, we have essentially lost our electrical roots. Our bare feet, with their rich network of nerve endings, rarely touch the ground. We wear insulating synthetic-soled shoes. We sleep on elevated beds made from insulating material. Most of us in the modern, industrialized world live disconnected from the Earth's surface. Although it is not something you probably have ever thought about, you may be suffering needlessly because of this disconnect. And you may be suffering severely, and in more ways than you could ever imagine.

As an analogy, think of a lightbulb with a loose connection. The bulb flickers, shines weakly, or doesn't light up at all. Many people go through life with flickering or weak health.

We believe this book is the first ever written about Mother Earth's natural "vibes" and how they keep us healthy and heal us—if we connect and stay connected to the source. Disconnected, the body seems vulnerable and prone to dysfunction, inflammation-related disease, and accelerated aging—a startling theory just beginning to gather scientific momentum.

This is the subject of our book.

The natural frequencies of the Earth that we speak of are waves of energy caused by the motions of subatomic particles called free electrons. Nobody has ever seen an electron, but you can think of them in the setting of a beehive. The bees, buzzing around the hive, are like electrons that move around the atomic nucleus in a "cloud" of energy. Another analogy used over the years is that of planets revolving around the sun. The nucleus contains protons, with a positive charge, and neutrons, that have, as their name implies, no charge. Electrons have a negative charge.

It is these electrons that give the Earth's surface a natural, negative charge. They are present, as science informs us, in a virtually limitless and continuously renewed supply, fed by the natural phenomena of rain and thousands of lightning strikes per minute. Maintaining contact with the ground allows your body to naturally receive and become charged with these electrons. When thus "grounded," you automatically absorb them, which in turn reduces electrical imbalances in the body and the oxidative free radicals involved in chronic inflammation and multiple diseases. The body's natural electrical state is restored.

This is the theory behind Earthing.

ELECTRICALLY CONDUCTIVE YOU

To understand the primordial relationship between bioelectrical you and your electrical planet, consider for a brief moment three types of materials used in electricity: conductors, insulators, and semiconductors. An example of a conductor is the metallic copper wiring in the walls of your house or in the electrical cord that you plug into an outlet from an appliance. The outer waves of electrons in conductors—corresponding in a simplistic way to the outermost bees buzzing around the beehive or to the distant planets orbiting around the sun—are so loosely bound that they easily move in the space between the atoms. They form a kind of gas around atoms and flow freely throughout the solid conductive material. That is why they are called free electrons. Think of them as free spirits, so to speak, not bound in a relationship with any atom composing the solid material.

In insulating materials, electrons are held in a tight grip by their atoms. There are no free electrons and consequently no current can flow through these materials. Examples of insulating materials include plastic, rubber, glass, and wood. You can now see why most of the time you are separated from the Earth. Your shoes' soles are made of plastic or rubber, and your house is made mainly of wood. Semiconductors are in between, sometimes conducting, sometimes not. Their electrical conductance is not as good as a conductor but not as bad as an insulator. Semiconductors are the backbone of modern electronic equipment because their conductance can be controlled by the application of an electric field.

Just like the Earth, your body is mostly water and minerals. Both are good conductors of electrons, and that's what makes you and the Earth electrically conductive.

Homo erectus, back a hundred thousand generations or so, didn't know a thing about any of this. Neither did the hunter-gatherers who followed in the human time line. Neither did the cultivator civilizations working the land about four hundred generations ago. And neither did the more recent Industrial Age incarnations. Even in today's electronic and wireless age, few know about the Earth's brimming reservoir of energetic free electrons.

Scientists back in the late 1800s first measured the Earth's subtle ground currents at different places around the world, using words such as "tranquil" and "quiet" to describe them. Present-day science refers to them as "telluric currents" and recognizes them as part of a larger system—called the "global electrical circuit"—involving clouds and the entire atmosphere. Geophysicists believe that this bank of almost limitless energy is continuously replenished with free electrons via an average of 5,000 lightning strikes per minute occurring perpetually around the planet. Without getting technical, the electrical potential present on the Earth's surface rises and falls according to the position of the sun. The intensity is more positive and energetic during the day, in support of your daily activities from wake up to shut down, and less positive and energetic during nighttime hours, promoting zzzzzzz. This daily high and low pattern sets in motion and orchestrates internal body mechanisms that regulate sleep-wake cycles, hormone production, and maintenance of health.

PAST CONNECTIONS

The basic phenomena of electricity were known since antiquity, but electricity was only harnessed for industrial and residential use about 120 years ago or so. The electron itself was discovered only in 1897, so virtually throughout the human time line nobody knew anything about electrons. But there was plenty of knowledge over the eons of time that the ground held special healing energy and was a basic aspect of connectedness to Nature. The Earth was sacred. This knowledge, passed down over countless generations, has survived in one form or another around the globe. Civilizations everywhere recognized and tuned in to the cycles of Nature for survival and health. They were aware of fundamental rhythms that regulate, for instance, sleep-wake cycles and maintenance of health, and they knew that we functioned in coordination with the Earth's cycles and rhythms. Awareness existed of connectivity among the principles of Earth, life, and health but expressed in the language of the day.

Qi (pronounced *chee*) is a central principle in the long history of Chinese knowledge and is regarded as the energy or natural force that fills the universe. From India's Vedic past comes an equivalent term, *prana*, meaning "vital force."

In the Chinese tradition, Heaven Qi is made up of the forces that heavenly bodies exert on the Earth, such as sunshine, moonlight, and the moon's effect on the tides. Earth Qi, influenced and controlled by Heaven Qi, is made up of lines and patterns of energy, as well as the Earth's magnetic field and the heat concealed underground. And within the Earth Qi, individuals, animals, and plants have their own Qi field. All natural things, in this concept, grow and are influenced by the natural cycles of Heaven Qi and Earth Qi.

Earth Qi is absorbed, without thinking about it, when we walk barefoot, which may explain why it's so relaxing to walk without shoes and why exercises geared toward strengthening the body and relaxing the mind (yoga, tai chi, and qigong, for instance) are often practiced without footwear. A central focus in Chinese practices involves "growing a root" and has to do with opening up communication between the bottom of the feet and the Earth. This process occurs through the "yong quan point," also known in acupuncture as the "kidney 1 point."

The ancient Greeks surely knew something about this concept. Hercules, one of the greatest heroes of Greek mythology, fought and defeated the giant Antaeus, who was renowned as a great wrestler. As the story goes, Antaeus was invincible as long as his feet remained in contact with the Earth, from where he drew his strength. He had never been defeated. Hercules, knowing Antaeus's secret, lifts the giant off the ground and strangles him to death.

Native Americans certainly honored the connection to the Earth. The late Ota Kte (Luther Standing Bear), a writer, educator, and tribal leader from the Lakota Sioux tradition, summed it up this way:

"The old people came literally to love the soil. They sat on the ground with the feeling of being close to a mothering power. It was good for the skin to touch the Earth, and the old people liked to remove their moccasins and walk with their bare feet on the sacred Earth. The soil was soothing, strengthening, cleansing, and healing."

CONNECT TO THE EARTH AND HEAL

This book will show you just how soothing, strengthening, and healing the Earth is. It will totally change the way you regard the ground under your feet and your relationship to the planet you live on.

For most people, reconnecting with Mother Earth usually means camping, hiking, gardening, going to the beach, or pursuing some other activity that returns us—in body and soul—to the bosom of Nature. The reconnection we talk about in this book is something different. By reconnection we mean taking off your shoes and socks and sitting, standing, or walking barefoot on the ground, something that is absolutely free and available (of course, where safe and comfortable). The reconnection can also involve the use of conductive bed sheets or floor mats linked by wire to a ground rod outside your house or office, or plugged into a wall outlet with a modern Earth ground system.

Either way, we call this reconnection process "Earthing" or "grounding," terms we will use interchangeably. They simply mean you are connected to Mother Earth. What you are doing is akin to what is well known in the electrical world as grounding, the common practice of connecting equipment and appliances to the Earth to protect against shocks, shorts,

"Vitamin G" for "Ground"

Exposure to sunlight produces vitamin D in the body. It's needed for health. Exposure to the ground provides "electrical nutrition" in the form of electrons. Think of these electrons as vitamin G—G for ground. Just like vitamin D, you need vitamin G for your health as well.

and interference. Applied to people, Earthing naturally protects the body's delicate bioelectrical circuitry against static electrical charges and interference. Most important, it facilitates the reception of free electrons and the stabilizing electrical signals and energy of the Earth. Earthing remedies an electrical instability and electron deficiency you never knew you had. It refills and recharges your body with something you never knew you were missing . . . or needed.

As you will read in this book, the results of Earthing often translate into a significant improvement—even total transformations—in health and vitality. One thirty-six-year-old woman with advanced multiple sclerosis (MS) was so happy about her improvement after Earthing that she once ran out of her house, stood in the middle of the street, and screamed to all her neighbors to get grounded. She said she wanted to start the "barefoot revolution" and teach everyone how to get well. She had tried Earthing out of desperation—something someone had told her about—after a doctor advised her to purchase an adjustable bed, a large screen television, and to make herself as comfortable as possible. MS doesn't get better, the doctor told her. In her case it did, and dramatically so.

Another woman spent over five years with debilitating pain, inflammation, fatigue, and sleep problems after a serious car accident. Despite a long career in the healthcare industry, she found herself locked in an exhausting struggle to regain her health. She went from one practitioner and treatment to another. "Like Humpty Dumpty in the nursery rhyme," she said, "all of the king's horses and all the king's men could not put me back together again." Unable to work, she found herself instinctively drawn to lying in the grass or walking barefoot on the beach. She began sleeping grounded and within months her pain, fatigue, and sleep problems vanished.

Even athletes, who operate at the most intense levels of physical human performance, have learned to ground and plug in to the natural energy of the Earth. From a group perspective, perhaps the most dramatic demonstration of Earthing's effectiveness occured at the Tour de France. The extreme physical and mental stress in this grueling race often causes sickness, tendonitis, and poor sleep among competitors. They tend to experience slow wound healing from accidents. In the 2003 to 2005 races, and again in 2007, American team cyclists were grounded after their daily competition. They reported better sleep, significantly less illness, practically no tendonitis, dramatic recovery from the day's racing, and faster healing of injuries. The practice has now been found to be so beneficial that other top athletes routinely Earth themselves.

Earthing is simple, basic, and powerful. We regard it as a genuine missing link in the health equation, something with astounding potential to do much good for humanity. Reconnecting to the Earth doesn't cure you of any disease or condition. What it does is to reunite you with the natural electrical signals from the Earth that govern all organisms dwelling upon it. It restores your body's natural internal electrical stability and rhythms, which in turn promote normal functioning of body systems, including the cardiovascular, respiratory, digestive, and immune systems. It remedies an electron deficiency to reduce inflammation—the common cause of disease. It shifts the nervous system from a stress-dominated mode to one of calmness and better sleep. By reconnecting, you enable your body to return to its normal electrical state, better able to self-regulate and self-heal.

In 1863, the eminent biologist T. H. Huxley stated that "the question of all questions for humanity, the problem which lies behind all others and is more interesting than any of them, is that of the determination of our place in nature and our relation to the cosmos." The content of this book explores that question from the simple perspective that your place in nature, in your immediate cosmos, requires you to be directly and routinely connected to the Earth under your feet.

In the pages ahead, we will explore the health implications of mankind's disconnect and present the unusual story about how the disconnect and the reconnect were discovered. You will read accounts of amazing healing from doctors and people from all walks of life. Most important, you will learn how easy it is to reconnect, to get Earthed, and to feel better.

CHAPTER 3

The Disconnect Syndrome

Illnesses do not come upon us out of the blue.
They are developed from small daily sins against Nature.
When enough sins have accumulated, illnesses will suddenly appear.
—HIPPOCRATES

The father of medicine clearly knew what he was talking about 2,500 years ago when he saw his Greek countrymen committing all kinds of sins against Nature. Imagine what he would think today just by looking at the most supposedly advanced country in the world. U.S. medical expenses, public and private, account for more than 17 percent of the gross national product and are projected to grow at a rate of 6 percent a year. By 2018, our medical bill will represent 20 percent of the country's earnings!

Ouch. That implies a lot of sickness and an inability of the medical system to prevent disease in the first place. Hippocrates would likely say there's a mighty amount of sinning going on.

In today's scientific age, an intense debate reverberates among researchers over what's to blame for the alarming increase in immune- and inflammation-related diseases.

In March 2008, an article by Rob Stein of the *Washington Post* brought attention to one of the primary issues responsible for the health meltdown: the decline of the human immune system. His article was entitled "Is Modern Life Ravaging Our Immune Systems?"

"First, asthma cases shot up, along with hay fever and other common allergic reactions, such as eczema," Mr. Stein wrote. "Then pediatricians started seeing more children with food allergies. Now experts are increasingly convinced that a suspected jump in lupus, multiple sclerosis, and other afflictions caused by misfiring immune systems is real.

"Although the data are stronger for some diseases than others, and part of the increase may reflect better diagnoses, experts estimate that many allergies and immune-system diseases have doubled, tripled, or even quadrupled in the past few decades, depending on the ailment and the country. Some studies now indicate that more than half of the U.S. population has at least one allergy."

Researchers blame modern living because the increases have shown up first largely in highly developed nations in Europe, North America, and elsewhere, and they are on the rise in other countries as they become more developed.

Globally, there's an "unprecedented rise" in diseases associated with inflammation and immune dysfunction, according to a 2012 report from the International Inflammation Network of researchers.

"Disturbing," said one French researcher, referring alone to the increase of autoimmune disorders, the difficult to treat and often disabling conditions stemming from a dysfunctional immune system that attacks the body's own cells, tissues, and organs. Common autoimmune diseases include lupus, rheumatoid arthritis, multiple sclerosis, and type 1 diabetes. The cause remains unknown, and the reasons for the increase are poorly understood. Collectively, they are among the most prevalent diseases in the United States, afflicting between 15 and 24 million people, about 75 percent of them women.

THE RISE OF INFLAMMATION

All these conditions—as well as the major disease killers like cardiovascular disease, type 2 diabetes, and cancer—are linked to chronic inflammation, a subject that has taken over center court in medical research during the last few years. As *Time* magazine reported in a 2004 cover article, "Hardly a week goes by without the publication of yet another study uncovering a new way that chronic inflammation does harm to the body." It torches the sensitive linings of the arteries that feed the heart and brain, leading to heart attacks and stroke. It chews up nerve cells in the brain and may contribute to the development of dementia and Alzheimer's disease. It can promote the proliferation of abnormal cells and facilitate their conversion into cancer. "In other words," the magazine said, "chronic inflammation may be the engine that drives many of the most feared illnesses of middle and old age."

The rise of inflammation in medical awareness has spawned a new term: "inflamm-aging." Italian researchers coined it in 2006 to describe a progressive inflammatory status and a loss of stress-coping ability as two major characteristics of the aging process.

Inflammation is now believed to be the underlying cause of more than eighty chronic illnesses, and more than half of Americans suffer currently from one or more of them. Each year, millions die from these conditions. The most common chronic diseases cost the U.S. economy alone more than $1 trillion annually—and that figure threatens to reach $6 trillion by the middle of the century.

"Inflammation may turn out to be the elusive Holy Grail of medicine— the single phenomenon that holds the key to sickness and health," wrote William Meggs, M.D., Ph.D., of East Carolina University in his book *The Inflammation Cure: How to Combat the Hidden Factor Behind Heart Disease, Arthritis, Asthma, Diabetes & Other Diseases* (2003).

THE MISSING LINK

Clearly, the contemporary immune system is being overwhelmed. The usual suspects in the scientific debate include genetics, poor diet, air pollution, obesity, physical inactivity, and even living in sterile homes. What has become evident to us is that researchers have overlooked another factor, something right under their noses, or to be more anatomically specific, right under their feet. In this book, we propose to add something new to the list of offenders: the lost connection to our planet's natural flow of surface electrical energy and the electron deficiency in our bodies this creates. Our investigations strongly suggest that the incidence of soaring chronic diseases during our lifetimes has occurred during a period in which more and more people have become increasingly disconnected from the Earth.

Is this disconnect and deficiency a missing link, an overlooked reason why sickness statistics rise ever higher? Is it perhaps the biggest cause of all? If inflammation is the Holy Grail of medicine, is connection to the Earth the Holy Grail of inflammation?

The answer to the first question is a resounding *yes.*

We don't presume to know yet the answer to the second and third questions. That will take years of investigation, but the initial research, along with many real life observations and experiences, provides intriguing evidence. This book is filled with that evidence. We believe that the information collected on the pages ahead packs the potential to reverse an alarming trend of failing health. We also think it can inspire entire new health standards and businesses based on reconnecting large segments of disconnected populations. We are sure that this information, if widely applied, can help any and all efforts to ease the healthcare burden shouldered by individuals, employers, and governments alike—literally from the ground up.

The evidence we have gathered strongly suggests that your health status stands to benefit in multiple ways when you reconnect, even if you are chronically and seriously sick and the medical system has little to offer you.

Throughout nearly all of our existence, the human immune system has provided protection for bodies living mostly in bare-skin contact with the Earth. We were naturally Earthed. Yet scientists haven't noticed that modern living involves a disconnect with Earth's stabilizing electrical energy and a loss of the body's natural grounded state, and that *this* loss may set up the immune system for malfunction.

Did the immune system—and the nervous system and other systems in the body—stop functioning properly when we began wearing shoes with insulating soles and living inside houses that insulate us from the natural frequencies of the environment?

Disconnecting Experimentally

What happens to the human body when it is separated from the subtle signals from the Earth was dramatically shown by experiments in Germany at the world-famous Max Planck Institute during the 1960s and 1970s. Researchers intentionally isolated volunteers for months at a time in underground rooms electrically shielded from the rhythms in the

Earth's electric field. Patterns of body temperature, sleep, urinary excretion, and other physiological activities were carefully monitored. All the participants developed a variety of abnormal or chaotic patterns, sort of like a head-to-toe arrhythmia. They experienced disturbed sleep and waking patterns, out-of-sync hormonal production, and overall a disruption in basic body regulation.

When electric rhythms comparable to those measured at the Earth's surface were pulsed into the metal shielding around the underground chambers, there was a dramatic restoration of normal physiological patterns.

These studies, involving hundreds of participants over many years, clearly documented the significance of the Earth's electrical rhythms for normal biological function. Normal rhythms in the body establish a stable reference point for repair, recovery, and rejuvenation—in short, for full health.

Clearly, the biological chaos induced in the experiments would lead in time to ill health. The conclusion is that the biological clock of the body needs to be continually calibrated by the pulse of the Earth that governs the circadian rhythms of all life on the planet.

Experiments like these, under controlled conditions, provide dramatic evidence. Yet we don't live underground. We live above the ground but not really on the ground—and that's the problem. We're disconnected. You can perhaps look at yourself and many people around you and get an idea of the consequences of this disconnect. There's a lot of sickness. Just read the health—rather, disease—statistics and you will see more evidence that in large or small part indicates a disconnect syndrome.

How are we disconnected even though we obviously live on the planet?

The Shoe Problem

Look at what you put on your feet on a daily basis. Most of you wear one form or another of footwear that evolved from simple foot coverings designed to protect against chilly and challenging ground conditions. You are likely wearing something much more elaborate, a statement reflecting your culture, fashion, behavior, and, in many cases, even identification with a tennis or basketball superstar. You habitually wear shoes even when they do not serve any practical purpose.

The late Dr. William Rossi, a Massachusetts podiatrist, footwear industry historian, prolific author, and keen observer, wrote many disturbing commentaries on what shoes do to our feet. He strongly believed that footwear is an integral part of foot care and often complained that shoe people didn't understand feet and foot-care people didn't understand shoes.

A "natural gait is biomechanically impossible for any shoe-wearing person," he wrote in a 1999 article in *Podiatry Management.* "It took four million years to develop our unique human foot and our consequent distinctive form of gait, a remarkable feat of bioengineering. Yet, in only a few thousand years, and with one carelessly designed instrument, our shoes, we have warped the pure anatomical form of human gait, obstructing its engineering efficiency, afflicting it with strains and stresses and denying it its natural grace of form and ease of movement head to foot."

Mechanical issues aside, Dr. Rossi was uncommonly attuned to the potential health risks caused by the separation of the Earth and the body created by modern shoes with soles made of insulating material.

"The sole (or plantar surface) of the foot is richly covered with some 1,300 nerve endings per square inch," he wrote in a 1997 article in *Footwear News.* "That's more than found on any other part of the body of comparable size. Why are so many nerve endings concentrated there? To keep us 'in touch' with the Earth. The real physical world around us. It's called 'sensory response.' The foot is the vital link between the person and the Earth. The paws of all animals are equally rich in nerve endings. The Earth is covered with an electromagnetic layer. It's this that creates the sensory response in our feet and in the paws of animals. Try walking barefoot on the ground for a couple of minutes. Every living thing, including human beings, draws energy from this field through its feet, paws, or roots."

Dr. Rossi referred to the foot "as a kind of radar-sonic base" providing a "little-known but vital function" that serves to "extract" energy from the Earth, similar to a plant root extracting moisture from the ground for nourishment. Such "ground-to-foot vibrations may thus be an important energizing power helping to serve the body's life forces," he suggested.

How right he was, even though he was mistaken in thinking that the source of this energy being drawn up into the body was magnetic. It is now well established that the energy residing on the surface of the Earth is primarily electrical. The central theme of our book is that we draw electrical energy through our feet in the form of free electrons fluctuating at many frequencies. These frequencies reset our biological clock and provide the body with electrical energy. The electrons themselves flow into the body, equalizing and maintaining it at the electrical potential of the Earth. Just like standard electronic equipment that needs a stable ground to function well, so, too, the body needs stable grounding to also function well.

Dr. Rossi bemoaned the fact that modern shoe soles have separated us from the energy and feeling of the ground, which is so important to the foot's sensory response. He wrote: "The bottoms of our footwear are vir-

The "World's Most Dangerous Invention"

David Wolfe, an author, nutritionist, speaker, and outspoken authority on health and lifestyle, deems "the common shoe" as perhaps the "world's most dangerous invention." After almost twenty years of lifestyle research, he incriminates the shoe as one of the "most destructive culprits of inflammation and autoimmune diseases" in our lives because it separates us from the healing energy of the Earth.

"Put a shoe on," he says, "and it's gone."

The Largest Medical Experiment Ever?

Marika Sboros, health news editor of *Business Day*, South Africa's leading business and financial daily, offered this perspective in a May 29, 2013, article:

"It's only since the Second World War that we have become disconnected from the Earth—literally—by wearing synthetic-soled shoes. The resultant insulation may represent the largest medical experiment ever undertaken, in which billions of people unknowingly participate every day. Who among us realizes that the massive, unintended consequences may be compromised health? One thing is for sure: The growth in immune/autoimmune-related diseases, especially cancer, has been staggering."

A Diabetes-Shoe Connection?

Refer to the chart "Correlation or Coincidence?" on page 85.

tually 'deadened.' A cross section of a shoe reveals several layers: outsole, midsole, insole filler material, footbed, cushioning, sockliner. An almost total blockout of sensory response."

Dr. Rossi's lament describes in a few words the post–World War II overhaul of shoe making. New materials entered the manufacturing scene: rubber, plastic, and petrochemical compounds. They have slowly squeezed out leather as the historical source of shoe soles. Nowadays, even makers of fancy men's dress shoes are increasingly switching to rubber, plastic, and other nonconductive material, just as casual and work shoes before them. Leather (processed from hides), a conductive material when moist, has been the traditional source of shoes and sandals. The original lightweight, softsole, heel-less and simple moccasin—a piece of crudely tanned leather that envelops the foot and is fastened on with rawhide thongs—is possibly the closest we have ever come to an "ideal" shoe. It dates back more than 14,000 years.

In his writings, Dr. Rossi also noted another intriguing connection between the foot and the ground—an erotic connection. The human foot, he wrote, is "rich with vibratory and electromagnetic powers linked to Earth contact—which is one reason for its age-old association with human fertility and the reproductive system."

The foot, he pointed out in his 1989 book, *The Sex Life of the Foot and Shoe* (Wentworth edition), is a primary sense organ lavishly equipped with "sexual nerves" and "every moment of standing or walking involves sensory contact with the ground." Erotic sensations "can be aroused by the touch of Earth, grass, wind, air, sun, sand, water. Such a sensation is experienced when you remove your shoes and stockings on a warm day and walk barefoot on the grass or sand, or dip your feet into a cool pool. The exhilaration is strongly sensual."

Beds and Beyond

For the most part, the modern structures we live and do business in—our homes and workplaces—are also nonconductive and separate us from the Earth's healing electrons. Think about where you spend most of your day: in an apartment, house, or office elevated off the ground, with a layer of wood, synthetic carpeting, or vinyl covering the floor. Unless you live on a dirt, cement, marble, or stone floor, it is unlikely that you are receiving any good vibes from below. We'll discuss later how living and working in multistory edifices may create a risk to health.

Like shoes and houses, beds, too, have evolved. They further separate most of us nowadays from the Earth for the third of the time we spend sleeping. We sleep (or toss and turn, as is the case for the masses of insomniacs) on nice and comfy padded elevated beds, in elevated houses, avoiding creeping and crawling things in the night.

The first record of raised beds is associated with the Egyptian pharaohs and their wealthy friends, thanks to the innovations of local Bronze Age craftsmen (3,000–1,000 B.C.). Although the fashion and the bedding has changed in the centuries since, the simple concept of sleeping on a platform resting on four legs hasn't changed much.

Before the Egyptians, however, humans apparently snuggled up for the night on the ground and, of course, where accessible, in nice, dry caves. Believe it or not, in this modern age there are still cave dwellers around, most notably 40 million or so in mountainous north-central China. They live surrounded by the Earth, and the Earth's energy, and, as we have heard, even with cable TV.

Anthropologists tell us they discovered evidence of grass-lined beds dating back over nine thousand years in southwest Texas. Pits were created in the soft sediment with grass piled in for some crude level of comfort. Whether straw, grass, or sleeping skins, these natural materials, when combined with perspiration from the body, have accommodated electron conductivity throughout the ages.

These are still the bedding materials of choice for many temperate-zone indigenous cultures around the world. Adult sleepers in traditional societies recline on skins, mats, the ground, or "just about anything except a thick, springy mattress," said a 1999 article at *Science News Online* that recommended researchers look at these societies for clues about sleeping patterns, insomnia, and nocturnal brain activity.

LIVING THINGS AS ANTENNAS

Our story brings us back to the transcendent question posed by T. H. Huxley about our relationship to Nature and the cosmos. In 1969, Matteo

Tavera, a French agronomist, put forward a unique answer in the form of a series of provocative hypotheses, contained in a largely unnoticed book, in which he argued that our place on the planet was to live in accordance with "natural electricity, which governs us all." Agronomy is the application of a combination of sciences like biology, chemistry, ecology, earth science, and genetics. Tavera's commentary, drawing from all these disciplines and many years of intimately observing Nature as a farmer, concludes that humans are paying a steep price in terms of degeneration and illness as a result of their separation from Nature.

Tavera's book, published in France under the title of *La Mission Sacrée* (*The Sacred Mission*), emphasizes the unrecognized electrical relationship of all living things—including plants, animals, and humans—to the ground and sky. The Frenchman saw life on the planet as being regulated by an energizing continuum from above and below, and that our structures were designed by Nature to receive and transmit that energy. Think of our bodies and forms as antennas, he said.

Tavera lamented that the modern lifestyle included "princely like structures, all built close together . . . with isolating floors, plastic clothing, and rubber-soled shoes. The electrical contacts are slowed down or totally missing" and, as a result, an increase in chronic illness has become quite evident.

Eating more wholesome food, free of chemicals, and breathing cleaner air certainly contributes to better health. But our "sacred, mission," he said, involves reconnecting with Mother Earth. Tavera warned that "man persists in going on in the direction of error," and while "Nature is forgiving, it has its limits to those who do not relate . . . and carry electricity through their bodies for the completion of the required health balance" necessary for survival.

The French naturalist said that humans should look at examples within the animal world to see why reconnection with Earth is so necessary. "Notice that a cow left in a stable with a more limited conduction of electricity due to the insulating effect of the building is usually cold and chilly," he wrote. "Put this same cow in the fields under the same weather conditions and it is quite comfortable. The cold nights are bearable. Chickens in the natural state of roaming never get sick. Chickens, isolated by their coop, need to be covered and protected . . . [and] look at the medicines that are required for the captive chicken. The quail in the wild have equal happiness in winter as in summer, without covering, without special lodging.

"The dog who is kept too long in the same habituation as his master and does not get to contact the Earth, as Nature intended, is keeping the veterinarian very busy.

"In the wild, the sanitary state of animals is excellent especially if it has not been soiled by the touch of man. Despite conditions seemingly uncomfortable to our eyes and probably because of those conditions, the wild animal knows no sickness. This privileged benefit is the result of his accomplishing his right to life by the proper exchange of the electric mediums.

"Be inspired by the wild animal [that] can survive so well on his own because of his constant contact with the Earth. Compare yourself to him a little."

Within the context of modern times, Tavera offered a variety of practical suggestions that could seemingly fit into most of our lifestyles. They included the following:

- "Walk into the wilderness and choose the grassy areas instead of the asphalt roads. Try to walk barefooted or at least with a covering that allows the electrical contact or exchange. You will notice the difference in your mood, your health. It will keep you alive with joy in your heart."

- "As often as possible expose any part of the skin of your body to the Earth or grass, or any natural water, lake, stream or ocean. In your garden . . . moist grass is a perfect conductor."

- "Use the trunk of a tree to lean on and rob it of some of its electricity for your health's benefit."

- "Bathing, especially in ocean water (because of the salts) or lake or river, is extremely good for you. If you can, walk barefoot in these waters. If you have ever done it you have already seen the benefits on your nervous system, your sleeping, your appetite, and your attitude. When you are linked to the Earth and involved in the electric exchanges, you start feeling like a human being again."

Matteo Tavera's writings are fascinating and alter the way one thinks about oneself, the environment, and our relationship with the cosmos. To read an English translation of his text on the Internet, visit the website www.earthinginstitute.net. His words offer great insight about our connectedness with Nature. What's even more fascinating is that the health implications raised by Tavera's commentary have been validated—not by a pedigreed scientist but by a nonscientist from the cable TV industry. His personal story follows next.

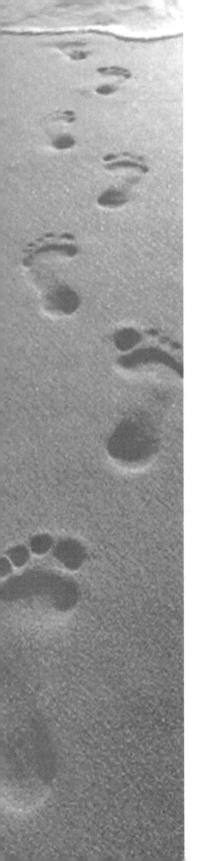

PART TWO

Personal Discoveries

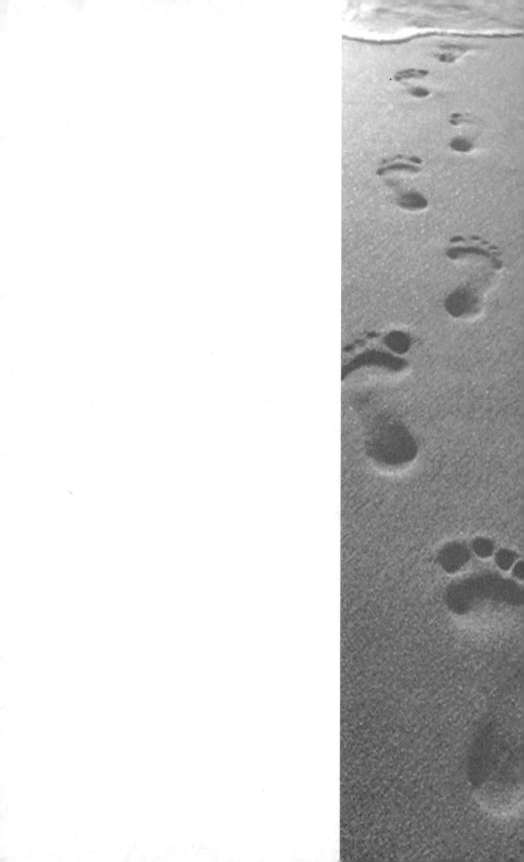

CHAPTER 4

Reconnecting:
Clint Ober's Story

In 1993, I was forty-nine years old, successful, and feeling on top of the world. I had come a long way from challenging and humble beginnings as a boy who grew up on a farm, chased cows, baled hay, and spent long summer days walking barefoot up and down long rows of beets and beans pulling weeds.

When I was a teenager, my father died of leukemia, leaving my mother and six children to tend the crops and livestock. Being the eldest son, I had to drop out of school and run the family farm. This was common practice back then under those kind of circumstances.

By the early 1960s, my brothers were getting older. I felt a need to leave the land for the excitement of the "big city." I wound up in the fledgling cable television industry. In the community I lived in, we only had two TV channels—one politically right, the other politically left, so the information we got was very slanted. I quickly saw that cable was the future of television. I jumped into it enthusiastically and had a lot of success organizing marketing campaigns to bring cable to people throughout Montana. I also climbed the poles, drilled the holes, sunk the ground rods, and ran the wire to install cable systems in many homes.

After a few years of working with local cable operators, I was hired as national director of marketing for a Denver company that soon grew to become the largest cable television operator in the United States. It was eventually acquired by AT&T. In 1972, I started my own business, specializing in developing cable television systems, as well as broadcast television and microwave communication properties. The company became the largest provider of cable television marketing and installation services in the country. We had a nationwide army of contract installers working for us. When a cable system was approved for some town or city, we'd send in ten to a hundred installers. They would go through the area and install everybody who wanted cable. Then they would go to the next town, and so on. Over the years we installed cable in millions of homes throughout the country.

In an age before the Internet, I helped pioneer the first-ever cable modem and distribution through personal computers of news reports from news agencies around the world. I also became intimately involved in the early development of programming and marketing for the cable and telecommunication industries. I worked with the top people who created Cable News Network (CNN), Home Box Office (HBO), and other cable networks.

I was a highly successful entrepreneur and living the good life. I had a 5,000-square-foot mountaintop home in Colorado with a 360-degree view of Denver and the Rockies. My house was full of art and anything that money could buy.

In 1993, the good life came tumbling down. I developed a serious abscess in my liver from a root canal procedure. Eighty percent of my liver was badly compromised. The infection had spread throughout my body. All my organs were malfunctioning. I didn't get much hope from the doctors. They suggested that I put my affairs in order.

However, one young surgeon told me there was a chance to survive—although a small one—involving experimental surgery to remove most of my damaged liver. He didn't give me much hope, but it was the only hope I had. So I agreed. After twenty-eight days of painful recovery in the hospital and much physical therapy, I was able to go home. I slowly began to regain my health. It took about three or four months to be able to walk a few blocks and six months to walk a mile. Amazingly, within nine months my liver grew back to its original size.

IN SEARCH OF A PURPOSE

One morning during my long mending process, I awoke and looked outside and noticed the sky was a deeper blue and the trees were a more vibrant green than I had ever seen before. At that moment, I felt alive again but very much different from before. A stark realization came over me that I didn't really own my home and the mountain of possessions I had. Rather, they owned me. My life had become all about taking care of my stuff. I'd spent my whole life accumulating, collecting, and taking care of it all, and trying to get more, perhaps to show off how big a success I was. I realized that I had become a slave to my possessions by my own making.

At that moment, I decided to set myself free and find something to fill my life with other than possessions. "I don't want anymore of this life," I said out loud to myself. "I want to do something different. Whatever time I have left I want to dedicate it to something worthwhile and with purpose."

I called my kids. They were all grown and scattered around the country. I told them to come and take whatever they wanted. "Anything you don't take, I'm going to give away," I said.

I sold the house. I sold the business to my employees. I went out and bought a recreational vehicle (RV), packed it up with a few necessities, and hit the road. I spent the next four years driving around the country, looking for myself and my mission. I spent a lot of time with my kids here and there, but a lot of time just doing nothing. I'd drive someplace and park for a while, waiting for something to show up.

One night in 1997 I was in Key Largo, Florida. I was getting antsy and impatient. Nothing was happening. Nothing was revealing itself to me. I had been in the same location now for a few months. While sitting and staring across the bay, I asked for guidance. I knew that something was waiting for me. When I returned to the RV, some words popped into my mind and I remember automatically writing them down on a piece of paper:

"Become an opposite charge."

Well, become an opposite charge to me meant to go out and poke people, and stir 'em up. Charge 'em up. I was sure getting impatient enough to do some stirring.

Then the second thing I wrote down was, "Status quo is the enemy." I didn't know what that meant except that I was getting tired of my status quo and doing nothing. That was the end of it. I wrote those thoughts down on a yellow tablet and kept it for some reason. I had no idea what those words really meant.

Upon rising the next morning, an odd notion went through my mind that the Earth itself was trying to tell me something. I didn't know what, though. But I felt there was some urgency, and I knew I had to go west somewhere for the answer. I drove to Los Angeles and felt it was too crazy. Then I drove to Tucson and Phoenix, and neither of those places felt right. So I headed north and wound up in Sedona at ten one night. I parked at a recreational vehicle resort by a creek. The next morning I looked out and was enchanted by the beauty of the land. The scenery spoke to my roots, of growing up in rural Montana, exposed to Native American culture that emphasized the connectedness to the natural world.

"I'm staying here," I told myself, "until I find what I'm looking for." So I stayed for almost two years. I made friends with many local artists and gallery owners. As a hobby, and to keep me busy, I spent a lot of my time artistically lighting up the town's many art galleries.

My "lightbulb" went off one day in 1998. I was sitting on a park bench and watching the passing parade of tourists from all over the world. At some point, and I don't know why, my awareness zeroed in on what all these different people were wearing on their feet. I saw a lot of those running shoes with thick rubber or plastic soles. I was wearing them as well. It occurred to me rather innocently that all these people—me included—were insulated from the ground, the electrical surface charge of the Earth beneath our feet. I started to think about static electricity and wondered if being insulated like that could have some effect on health. I didn't know the answer, one way or another. The notion just popped into my mind.

I thought back to my years in television and cable. Before there was cable, you commonly had lots of flecks ("noise," we call it) in the TV picture. Or you had "snow" or lines and all kinds of electromagnetic interference. If you aren't old enough to remember that, you are likely familiar with the radio interference when you're driving near or under a power line and you hear all that crackle and pop.

In the cable industry, you have to ground and shield the entire cable system in every home to prevent extraneous electromagnetic signals and fields from interfering with the transmission carried through the cable.

That's how you provide the viewer with a perfect signal and a crisp picture, as well as preventing signals on the cable system from leaking out into the environment and possibly disturbing police radio or TV station transmissions. The cable consists of an inner copper conductor, an insulating layer, and an outer shield. The shield is electrically connected to the Earth. It is grounded, so that the Earth can either deliver or absorb electrons and prevent damage from electrical charges. All of the cable system must be grounded and held at the same electrical potential as the Earth's surface.

What Is Electrostatic Discharge?

Static electricity is nothing more than the spark or minor shock we all experience, for instance, when we touch a metal doorknob after walking across a carpeted room (see figure below) or slide across a car seat. No big deal.

But in some industries, it is a very big deal. Centuries ago, armed forces had to use static control measures to prevent ignition of gunpowder stores. Today, such measures are required in the petroleum industry, where a random spark can also cause an explosion. In today's electronic industry, electrostatic discharge (ESD) causes billions of dollars in damage annually by destroying highly sensitive electronic parts and microchips. ESD affects production yields, manufacturing costs, product quality, product reliability, and profitability.

A whole static control industry has emerged with products such as wristbands, shoes, and conductive flooring that are widely used by electronics makers. These measures are designed to discharge potentially destructive charges.

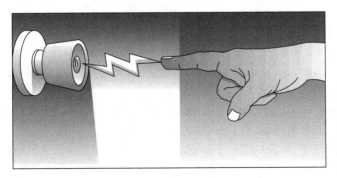

Finger to the doorknob, showing electrostatic discharge.

THE BEGINNING OF AN ADVENTURE

Little did I know at the time, but my life was about to take a new and totally unexpected direction that would consume practically all my waking hours. It still continues to do so, a dozen years later.

It all started innocently with that one simple question: Could wearing rubber- or plastic-soled shoes, as we all do, and insulating ourselves from the ground, affect health? At the time I had a particular interest in health because earlier back surgeries had left me with constant back pain. I never slept well. I'd take Advil to go to bed, and in the morning I'd take Advil to get up and get through the day. I also took other pain medication, depending on how bad the pain was.

I knew that the body was conductive, that is, it conducts electricity. You don't have to know anything about electricity to understand that simple fact of life. Just go touch a doorknob on a very dry day and you can see or feel a spark every time. There's always a static charge on the body that builds up when you sit on fabric-covered furniture or walk on carpets.

An Amazing Experiment

Sitting there watching the foot traffic I realized that most people, certainly in the industrialized world, had little or no connection to the ground. In other parts of the world, like in the tropics and in Asia, Africa, and South America, rural people walk barefoot and often sleep on the ground. They are grounded.

I decided to try to answer the question I had asked myself. I went back to the apartment I was renting and picked up my voltmeter. (A voltmeter is an instrument that measures the electrical potential differences between the Earth and any electrical object, or any two points in an electrical circuit.) I connected a 50-foot wire to it and ran the wire out the living room door and attached it to a simple ground rod I stuck in the Earth. Then I started walking around the house and measuring the electrical charges being created on my body from being insulated from the ground. It was easy to measure the static electricity, as it would vary with every step that I took. What I found most interesting was the amount of electromagnetic field (EMF) induced potential (in volts) on my body. When I walked toward a lamp, the voltage would go up. When I stepped back, the voltage went down. I tested this with all the electrical appliances in the living room and kitchen. The only appliances that did not create EMF voltage on my body were the refrigerator and my computer tower. They were grounded. From my background in the communications industry, this immediately made sense to me as we had to ground all of our electronic equipment to prevent electrical interference from EMFs.

Next I went to the bedroom, lay down on my bed, and registered the highest level of EMF voltage on my body. The bedroom was the most "electrically active" area of the apartment. The bed was up against a wall full of hidden electrical wires. I wondered if these electric fields could be affecting my ability to fall asleep because sleep was always a big problem.

Now my curiosity was really stirred up. The next day I went to the hardware store and bought some metallized duct tape that is used for furnace ducting. I laid some of that tape out on the bed to form a crude kind of grid. I took an alligator clip and attached it to one end of the duct tape grid. I connected a wire to it, ran the wire out the window, and fastened it to another ground rod similar to the one that the voltmeter was connected to. I then lay down on the duct tape grid and noticed that the meter was now showing nearly zero, meaning that I was in sync, that is electrically equivalent, to lying directly on the ground outside. Like all the cable systems I had installed, I was physically grounded. I was lying there fooling around with the voltmeter and the next thing I knew it was morning. I had fallen asleep with the voltmeter on my chest. I hadn't needed a pill to fall asleep. I had slept soundly for the first time in years, and I had hardly moved at all during the night.

"Wow, this is fascinating," I said to myself. Something interesting had happened, but I didn't really understand the meaning of it. So I repeated this experiment on myself the next night. I fell asleep without a pill. The same thing happened the next night and the next and the next.

Getting High Off the Ground

After a few more days like this, I told a couple of friends about it and asked them if I could set up a similar kind of makeshift grid with metallic duct tape in their beds. That's how I started "grounding" people. It was very innocent. One of the guys I grounded said to me, "You know, something is going on here. My arthritis pain is way down."

I didn't think too much about what he said, but a couple of days later I noticed that my own severe chronic pain had improved. I didn't need the pain pills anymore. I was also feeling much better overall.

I didn't understand anything about biology. I didn't understand how the nerves or muscles worked, but a concept was dawning. It occurred to me that there might be an analogy between the human body and cable TV. Cable has hundreds of channels of information flowing through it. Similarly, the body has countless nerves, blood vessels, and other channels that conduct electrical signals. Maybe, I thought, when the body is grounded, it prevents the entry of "noise"—environmental electrical interference—that could disturb the internal circuitry. I started to understand in a simple way that without Earth contact the body was always being charged by the electromagnetic fields and static electricity in the bedroom or office or wherever. When you're grounded, you don't have a charge. When I grounded myself and my friends, the charges were removed, and we all started sleeping better and feeling better.

After I grounded a half dozen or so people, consistently improving their sleep and reducing their pain, I started to get a real high. I became more and more excited. I came to the conclusion that I may have made a great discovery. I said to myself there's something very, very real here that needs to be further investigated.

I looked far and wide but didn't find much information on grounding and health. In 1999, the Internet wasn't nearly the information universe it is today. It was still fairly new and I didn't find anything there.

I checked out the excellent university medical libraries in Arizona but didn't come up with anything. There were a few anecdotal stories about Native Americans that were folklorish in nature. I was reminded of my younger days in Montana where many of my childhood friends were kids from the Indian reservation. I vividly remembered the time when the sister of one of my friends developed a bad case of scarlet fever. She was very sick. Their grandfather dug a pit in the ground and placed the girl in the pit. He built a fire, for warmth, near the pit, and sat next to it for a few days while the girl mostly slept. At the end of that time she was much better. I also remembered going to the home of one of my friends after school and hearing his mother tell him to remove his shoes. "They will make you sick," she said. This all seemed very odd to me at the time, but I remembered that most things the Native Americans did were different from what I was taught to be normal. I later realized that there was always a reason based on much greater knowledge of Nature than I was ever taught.

I found information about barefoot enthusiasts who have long championed the idea of going unshod because they feel better. Some enthusiasts have formed organizations, such as the worldwide Society for Barefoot Living that promotes the benefits of taking shoes and socks off and walking naturally on the Earth. Their experience, along with medical research in the field of biomechanics, strongly suggests that many foot and back problems are partly caused by stresses and strains created by wearing shoes that force us to stand and move in ways the human body was not designed for. One dramatic example of this appears to be the success of barefoot runners. The shod foot may explain the high injury frequency in North American runners, in contrast to the extremely low running-related injury frequency in barefoot populations. Researchers have found, for instance, less force on the joints, and less plantar fasciitis and shin splints. This, however, wasn't really the information I was looking for.

I did find considerable information about electrostatic discharge and how people working on computer components and electronic chips had to be grounded in order not to damage any of the components electrically. But that wasn't it either. I had to keep looking.

I also wanted to know whether there was any possibility that sleeping "Earthed," as I started to call grounding, could be harmful. Electronics experts reassured me that the concept was perfectly safe. If you think about it, being Earthed is the natural state of living systems throughout history. It is the separation from Earth that is unnatural.

Beyond these few things, however, I couldn't uncover any concrete information anywhere relating to the possible health effects due to loss of natural grounding.

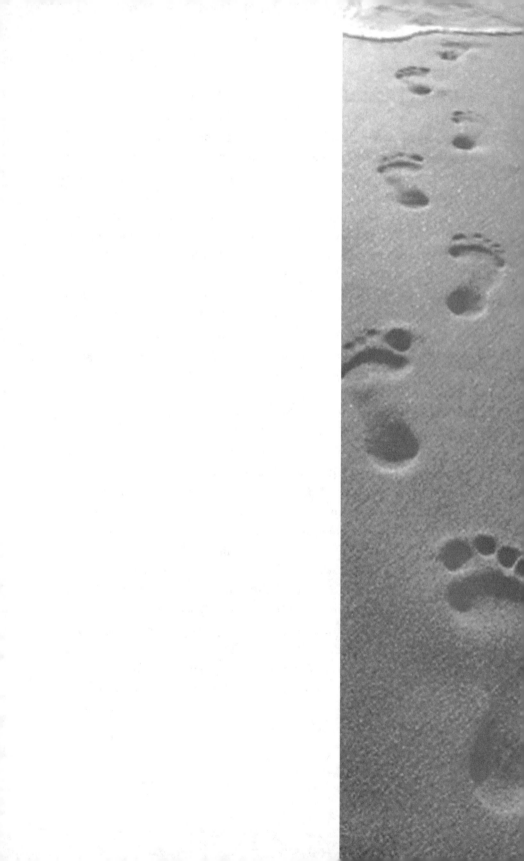

CHAPTER 5

Challenges of
an Amateur Scientist

E motionally, I was on a roller coaster. I came to the conclusion that nobody—past or present—had researched the grounding/health connection. I couldn't find any relevant information. When I realized that nobody else knew about it, I felt like it was the best day in my life and that I had discovered something important with which to help society in a big way. I had found my mission. And I was the only one who knew anything about it.

The euphoria didn't last long. Maybe that's the way it is with discoveries. The self-doubt starts to creep in that comes from being alone with some important understanding or breakthrough before anybody accepts your idea.

In my case, anybody I talked to thought I was nuts. Nobody took me seriously. Nobody knew anything. My enthusiasm would always be returned by blank stares of indifference or negative responses. Who said this was so? People wanted hard facts. They wanted science. I was just an ex-cable guy talking about how the ground could reduce your pain and let you sleep better. What did I know? What credentials did I have?

So I went quickly from the best day in my life to the worst day. I was feeling down in the dumps one day in 1999 as I was sitting and talking with one of the guys in Sedona whom I'd grounded. He was telling me how good he felt and how big the change was in his life. Hearing him say those words reignited a spark and lifted my spirits.

I said to him, "I'm feeling good from this, too. Other people are telling me the same thing. This is real. I'm not making anything up. There's no ifs, ands, or buts about it. I've just got to find the answers."

With new resolve, I packed up and drove to California in my RV, an amateur detective trying to solve a mystery. I figured I'd spend a few months out there and hopefully turn up some real expertise that I could tap into, some people to teach me more, or to figure out how to quantify what all this was about.

"STRANGER IN A STRANGE LAND"

The first thing I did was try to interest sleep researchers in Southern California. I made phone calls. I knocked on doors. I introduced myself as a guy with an electrical background who has made some interesting observations about sleep and pain. I had seen dramatic results. I said I wanted to get some experts to validate my observations.

In pursuit of expertise, I felt like the hero of Robert Heinlein's old science fiction classic, *Stranger in a Strange Land*. I felt I was on another planet. I didn't speak the language. They didn't speak mine.

Imagine how I felt walking into the office of a scientist or doctor, if I got that far. The office walls were full of awards and diplomas. These were individuals who had spent years becoming experts in their field. And here I was, with absolutely no formal training in the field. The experts used biological terms I never heard of. When I would turn the conversation to electrical concepts that I understood, like voltages, electric fields, grounding, and positive and negative charges in the body, they were about as clueless as I was hearing them talk about what they knew.

Communication was just one problem. Another was that most scientists or doctors had no desire to get involved or lend their name to anything out of left field like this, something with no scientific history or legitimacy.

One scientist sat back and laughed in my face. He asked if I expected him "to believe that sticking a nail in the ground and connecting it to an iron bed pad and getting people to sleep on it will reduce pain." He said he wouldn't believe it even if it were published in the *New England Journal of Medicine*.

One doctor told me that, even if what I was saying were true, why should he tell patients to take off their shoes and get well for free?

Another stated that I needed to provide him with all the published research related to grounding the body and he would then take a look at it. When I told him there was no research and that is why I was approaching him, he said to come back after someone substantiates the validity of grounding.

One amused researcher asked if I had any idea about what it takes to do research. He told me it would take five years and $5 million to put together a real scientific study and get it published, if it even got that far.

Most of the experts I spoke to were polite, but nobody took any interest. They sent me on my way and wished me good luck. That's when I decided to do the first study myself.

GETTING THE SCIENCE BALL ROLLING

All wasn't lost though. At one university sleep clinic, I managed to talk to some friendly students. They said they would be willing to counsel me on how to do a study. I didn't have a clue. One thing I had to figure out was how I could ground people for any length of time, long enough so that I could identify a measurable result. People are always moving around. They are busy.

So I went back to my own experience. The only way to do this, I realized, was when somebody was in bed, at night, when sleeping. That's the only time people are still. That seemed to be the most practical way to produce a measurement. So a bed pad of some sort seemed the best way to go. But I had to design something more substantial than the crude metallic duct tape grid I was using for myself and friends.

I contacted a company that makes protective equipment for the electronics industry. I had some special conductive fiber materials manufactured that I then bonded to 1-by-2-foot wool felt pads. The test subjects were to sleep directly on the pad placed on their bed. I fixed a metallic snap on each pad so I could connect it to a wire running to a ground rod stuck in the Earth outside the bedroom window. Now that I had a pad, I needed people for the experiment.

As you can imagine, no doctors would lend me patients for my little study. I was on my own. I got the inspiration for volunteers one day while getting my hair cut. I heard people in the salon talking about their health issues. I figured that a beauty salon could be a good source of volunteers.

I convinced the woman who operated the salon to try grounding first. I set her up with a grounded bed pad. Her feedback was positive. She was sleeping better. She enthusiastically approached some of her clients to participate in the study. I found others by leaving fliers in ten beauty shops in Ventura, California, where I was living at the time.

One of the people who stepped forward was a nurse. She was a great help, smoothing the way so I could enter the homes of strangers, explain the bed pads, actually place them in people's beds, and connect them to simple ground rods I stuck in the Earth outside their bedroom windows. What I was doing was not exactly your ordinary house call. In the end, I was able to enroll sixty people—thirty-eight women and twenty-two men—with sleep problems and a variety of joint and muscle pain.

Based on the advice I had received from the sleep clinic students, I divided the volunteers into two groups. Half slept on pads that were actually grounded. For comparison, the other half slept on bed pads that looked like they were connected to the ground rods, but I inserted a spacer on the wire to block conduction. The volunteers did not know if they were actually connected or not. I was the only one who knew.

The nurse interacted with the people during the thirty days' experiment. Then she collected the data. We then wrote up the experiment as an anecdotal study and published it in 2000 on *ESD,* an online journal that provides articles, technical papers, news items, and book reviews on the subject of electrostatic discharge.

The results were extraordinary. Here is what we found afterward when we compared the grounded group with the ungrounded one:

- 85 percent went to sleep more quickly.

- 93 percent reported sleeping better throughout the night.

- 82 percent experienced a significant reduction in muscle stiffness.

- 74 percent experienced elimination or reduction of chronic back and joint pain.

- 100 percent reported feeling more rested when they woke up.

- 78 percent reported improved general health.

Several participants reported unexpected but significant relief from asthmatic and respiratory conditions, rheumatoid arthritis, hypertension (high blood pressure), sleep apnea, and premenstrual syndrome (PMS). There were also reports of fewer hot flashes.

Discovery of the "Magic Pain Patch"

One woman who participated in the study had crippling rheumatoid arthritis in the joints of her hands and arms, and she had difficulty walking. I wanted to measure how much electrical charge she had on her body in her bedroom and asked her to hold a small, handheld tester for me. She couldn't. Her arthritis was too severe and too painful. So in order to get a reading I adhered an electrode patch—the same kind used by doctors when they do EKG (electrocardiogram) tests—on her forearm and connected it with an alligator clip to the ground wire coming into her bedroom. I then connected and disconnected the clip in order to read the change in the body charge between being grounded and ungrounded. After chatting for five or ten minutes while I was setting up the bed-pad system, the woman said the pain in her arm improved considerably. She then asked me to move the patch to her other arm. I did not believe what she was saying, but I did what she asked and moved the patch to the other arm. Minutes later, she said the pain in that arm had gone down a good deal as well.

After leaving her home, I immediately called several acquaintances I knew who had arthritis and other painful conditions and gave them each setups with electrode patches, Earthing wires, and ground rods. I wanted to see if I could repeat this dramatic reduction of localized pain. Remarkably, each and every one of them reported a rapid reduction in pain. A couple of them referred to it as the "magic pain patch." This is when I first discovered that localized Earthing of the body in this manner produced fast and dramatic reduction of local pain. It was kind of like pouring water on a fire.

Now I was really excited. I felt encouraged. But still no scientists would talk to me seriously about it. My student buddies told me that I needed to produce much more solid information to support my idea. Anecdotal studies wouldn't be enough, they said, and wouldn't stand up to scientific scrutiny.

Refining the Discovery

Initially I regarded the positive results I was witnessing as a consequence of eliminating static electricity and/or the shielding of the body from environmental electric fields. This assumption turned out to be absolutely true, but accounted only in part for all the good results.

When I installed the Earthing system in people's homes for the first study, I always measured their body voltages while they were lying in bed—both before and after placing the grounding pad on the bed. When I measured people with extremely high body voltage, I would think to myself that I should get some really good results from this person.

One day I set up a volunteer, a sixty-five-year-old man, who complained of chronic pain and problems with sleeping. He had no electrical devices near the bed. His floor was bare concrete. When I measured his body voltage, it registered near zero. With very little body voltage, I thought we wouldn't get any results from him. However, his feedback in the end was as good as others with high body voltages.

His case was the first indication I had that Earthing alone produced the results that I myself had experienced and observed in others. This realization stopped me in my tracks. I then had to learn everything I could about the Earth's electrical properties.

I learned, for instance, that the Earth's electrical surface charge is always negative, meaning that the surface is filled with free electrons. They are able to move and reduce a positive charge. In Nature, lightning is the best example of a negative charge reducing a positive charge.

If Earthing people reduces their chronic pain, that suggested to me that pain is related to positive charge. I then began to ground people in low- or no-electric field environments to replicate this observation and confirm that it was the grounding alone that reduced pain. The results were consistent. Earthing reduced pain no matter what the electrical environment. It wasn't until later that I learned the connection between chronic pain and inflammation, and the role of electrons.

NORMALIZING THE HORMONE OF STRESS

When the first study was published, it created a big stir among researchers and health practitioners concerned about the health risks from exposure to environmental electric fields. One such person I met at this time was Maurice Ghaly, a retired anesthesiologist in Southern California who was interested in electric field research. I told him what I had learned. He pretty much dismissed my theory. But he said he would like to prove me wrong. It didn't make sense to him that grounding could do what I said it did.

Dr. Ghaly decided on a pilot study. He would measure the circadian secretion of cortisol on people before and after they slept grounded, over a period of a few weeks. Cortisol is known as the "stress hormone." When you become worried, fearful, and anxious, your cortisol level rises. The rise stimulates a branch of the autonomic nervous system known as the sympathetic system. Your body shifts into a vigilant mode, ready, if needed, to fight or run, the so-called fight-or-flight mode. The hormone level comes back down after the vigilance and tension ease. A life of constant stress—from common things like money, work, or relationship problems—also causes your cortisol level to rise and remain high, creating a kind of sympathetic overdrive in the body. In our day and age, a consistently high level is a classic indicator of stress and is known to contribute to many health problems, like sleep disorders, hypertension, cardiovascular disease, reduced immune response, autoimmune disease, mood disturbances, and blood sugar irregularity. Stress of this kind also promotes inflammation in the body.

My first study was subjective, based on the feedback of people I grounded. This time we would measure a substance produced in the body, thus providing an objective measurement for the effect of Earthing on the physiology. It was a big step forward scientifically.

For the study, I needed something that would hold up even better than the previous bed pad. So I designed a sturdier bed pad that would fit over the whole mattress.

We enrolled twelve subjects who complained of sleep problems, pain, and stress. They slept on the Earthing pads I made up for eight weeks. Their individual daily cortisol levels were determined at four-hour intervals over a twenty-four hour period just before the start of the study and then once again at the three-quarter mark via a standard saliva test. The participants also reported daily how they were feeling throughout the entire experiment.

The study was published in a 2004 issue of the *Journal of Alternative and Complementary Medicine*. The conclusion was significant: Earthing during sleep resynchronizes cortisol secretion more in alignment with its natural, normal rhythm—highest at 8:00 AM and lowest at midnight. Figure 5-1 provides a visual representation of the dramatically improved cortisol group profile.

Subjectively, the participants reported improved sleep along with reduced pain and stress. Even more impressive was the fact that the improvements often occurred within the very first days of sleeping grounded.

Following is a summary of the findings:

• All but two subjects developed more natural cortisol rhythm, and one of the exceptions was someone already in a normal pattern.

• Eleven of twelve participants said they fell asleep faster.

Cortisol levels before and after grounding

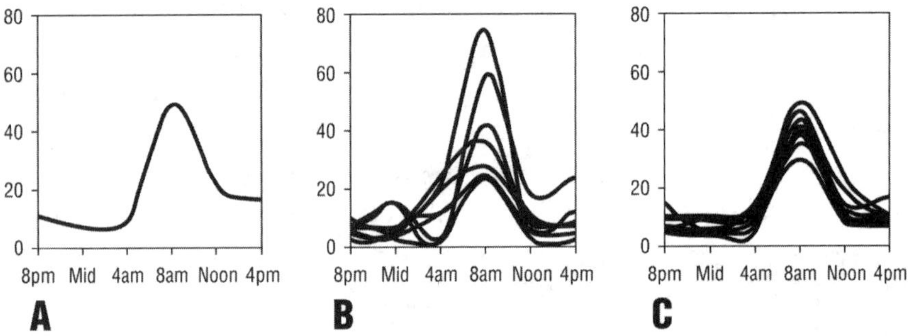

Figure 5-1. Realignment of natural cortisol rhythms.
In unstressed individuals, the normal twenty-four-hour cortisol secretion profile follows a predictable pattern—lowest around 12:00 midnight and highest at 8:00 AM (Graph A). The pregrounding chart (Graph B) shows the wide variation of patterns among the study participants. Graph C represents the altered pattern of the participants after Earthing, showing a significant stabilization of cortisol levels. Seven participants registered a reduction in high- to out-of-range nighttime cortisol secretion, a 53.7 percent average drop; six had an average rise toward normal of 34.3 percent in 8:00 AM levels; and two with abnormally high 8:00 AM levels had an average drop of 38 percent. (Data adapted from *The Journal of Alternative and Complementary Medicine*, 2004.)

- All twelve reported waking fewer times during the night (from an average of 2.5 times to 1.4 times, a 44 percent reduction).

- Nine out of twelve said they felt more refreshed and less fatigued, with more daytime energy, while three reported no change.

- Of the eleven subjects who said before grounding that their pain interfered with general activities, seven now reported improvement and only four said there was no change.

- Nine out of twelve described reductions in their emotional stress and were less bothered by problems such as anxiety, depression, and irritability; two said there was no change; one said the stress was worse.

- Six out of seven participants with gastrointestinal symptoms reported improvements.

- Five out of six women with either PMS and/or hot flashes said their symptoms were better,

- All three individuals with TMJ (temporomandibular joint) pain said their discomfort was less.

The Sleep Connection

The study produced another quite interesting finding that was not published but provided more evidence about the multiple benefits of Earthing. Eight of our participants had an increase in melatonin ranging from 2 to 16 percent. Three subjects had no change in their melatonin level, and one experienced a decrease of 6 percent. The finding was exciting because melatonin is an important hormone that helps regulate sleep and other biological rhythms and is also a powerful antioxidant agent with anticancer properties.

Right from the start of my experimenting with Earthing—and by right from the start I mean my own initial experience—the positive impact on sleep has been very noticeable. This is a big deal. We all need good rest to allow our bodies to repair and recover from each day's activities. That's the way Nature set things up: cycles of rest and activity.

After I saw how grounding was helping people sleep, I started to research the sleep problem. I found a 2002 *Newsweek* article entitled "In Search of Sleep" that said there were an estimated 70 million problem sleepers in the United States alone. "I Can't Sleep" was the title of a *Businessweek* cover story in 2004. From those, and many other sleep-related articles from all over the world, it became quite clear to me that quality sleep improves overall health and that poor sleep does just the opposite.

I also learned that back in the early 1970s researchers identified several behaviors that were positively linked to length of life. Sleep headed the list, followed by exercise, eating breakfast, and avoiding snacks. Weight, smoking, and moderating alcohol intake also made the list. Later on, researchers found that sleep deprivation may enable bacterial growth and that sufficient sleep may slow down bacterial growth. More recently, sleep deprivation—even a modest reduction—was found to promote inflammation in the body. Loss of sleep, even for a few short hours during the night, apparently prompts the immune system to turn against healthy tissue and organs. Other new studies suggest that sleep loss may also contribute to recurrent depression.

In my ongoing sleuthing, I learned that since the pioneering research in the 1950s of Hans Selye, the father of stress medicine, medical researchers believe there is a relationship between imbalances in cortisol and inflammatory pain.

It was becoming clearer and clearer to me that Earthing was something very special that could make people's lives better in a multitude of ways. It was this vision that kept me going, because there were many times when I frankly felt overwhelmed by the challenge of me—an unknown quantity with no degree by my name, or even a high school education—proving a totally foreign concept to the scientific community.

MORE CHALLENGES: BEDS, SPOUSES, AND FASHION

My first sleep study created a buzz when it was published in 2000. I was hounded by people wanting bed pads. All of a sudden, there was a demand for this "quasi product." I didn't realize it at the time, but I was becoming somewhat of a designer of Earthing pads. Later, when I got involved in Earthing people in the world of sports, athletes didn't want a whole bed pad. It was too much to carry around. They wanted something they could roll up and put in a small bag and take with them when they traveled. Thus, the recovery bag was born: conductive silver strands woven into cotton sheets fitted together like a sleeping bag.

The products developed both out of a demand by people who heard about Earthing as well as a desire on my part to promote scientific research. It all started on an ad-lib basis with conductive duct tape and a wire connection to a ground rod. That's what I used in Arizona on myself, friends, and other interested people. It was all makeshift. Nothing sophisticated.

As this evolved, people simply wanted something more refined. Some people wanted sheets, so I started consulting with experts in the fabric industry. I first dabbled in polyester with carbon threads. But nobody wanted polyester, so I switched to cotton with conductive silver strands. That development cost more than $1 million and took three to four years. I first had to find manufacturers to deal with what for them was a nuisance factor, and then test and retest. These were all prototype products that cost a lot of money to make, and, for the most part, I was giving them away to athletes, doctors, and people in the studies and their relatives. It all mushroomed. I would get rid of one model, then order more, then get another batch of new material, and then another flurry of orders and requests. I never for a moment thought I would be in the sleeping or bedding industry.

In the early days, a lot of doctors started getting products for their patients. One of them called and asked if I had some kind of a "half pad," a sheet that didn't cover the whole bed. I asked why he wanted it. He referred to the spouse problem.

Spouse problem?

Here is what was going on: If a woman got a bed pad, the husband would get upset and say he didn't want anything to do with this, that it was just a waste of money. If the husband brought it home, the woman would say this is crazy and get it off her side of the bed.

Throughout this time, the mode of the day was to put sheets on your bed with the highest possible thread count. The buzz was 300-, 600-, 1,200-, and then 2,400-count sheets. The higher the count, the more luxurious, softer, and finer the fabric is supposed to be. This concept became very popular, but some experts think that higher thread counts simply mean a higher price tag.

Anyway, I got caught up in this. If you had anything else but high thread count on your bed, you were not in fashion. Then there was the issue of designer colors to match décor and color tastes. In a typical marriage, nothing goes on a bed without a woman's permission. So you couldn't put just anything on a bed—no matter what the health benefits.

I didn't need these kinds of extraneous issues. One day I decided to just make a half sheet that could be placed across the width of the bottom of the bed. You make contact with it with your feet, like putting your feet on the Earth, and this is your barefoot connection. The half sheet could also be used lengthwise on one side if a spouse didn't want to have anything to do with it.

The half sheet solved a lot of my headaches, as well as reducing the pain level for many people who slept on them.

CHAPTER 6

A Cardiologist's Discovery: Steve Sinatra's Story

As an integrative cardiologist, I use both conventional and alternative medicine to help my cardiac patients. This approach has always worked superbly for me as a doctor and, above all, for my patients, because it focuses on the metabolic operation of cells and particularly the cells in the heart muscle that pump blood throughout the sixty thousand miles of blood vessels in the body. As such, I have used many excellent nutritional supplements, like coenzyme Q_{10} (CoQ_{10}), carnitine, and magnesium, to boost the metabolic processes in the cells where energy production takes place.

Years ago, after a decade or so in practice, I slowly became aware of a curious pattern: increased patient complaints—notably arrhythmias and chest pain (angina)—around the time of a full moon or intensified solar flare activity. I don't remember how I actually connected the symptoms with celestial events—it may have been a patient who said something. I certainly had no real clue how to explain it. In any case, my curiosity was tweaked and I began looking for information, which led me into the amazing world of electromedicine.

The term may sound way out in left field and conjure images of Dr. Frankenstein, Dr. Sivana, Goldfinger, and otherworldly contraptions that snap, crackle, and pop. However, electromedicine is quite an accepted concept, most obviously for diagnostics that include everyday medical tools such as EKGs and MRIs (magnetic resonance images). Less accepted, but gaining increased medical attention and respect, are electromagnetic treatment devices such as pulsed electromagnetic field units to address pain and musculoskeletal disorder. Pain-reducing TENS (transcutaneous electrical nerve stimulation) machines, utilizing low electrical voltage, have been around for many years.

My research and conversations with experts has given me a growing understanding as to how electromagnetic events going on in the heavens or right here on the planet can have a response—positive or negative—on the heart, the brain, and the rest of the body. For sure, we terrestrials are not isolated from the rest of the universe and are subject to influences ranging from galactic and solar forces down to local, man-made electricity and electronics.

All beings are conglomerations of bioelectrical energy. In essence, our bodies function—for better or for worse—as a collection of dynamic electrical circuits.

One of the primary electrical entities in the body is the heart. Each beat is triggered by an electrical signal from within the heart muscle, activity that is recorded when you undergo an EKG in your doctor's office. Each signal, repeated nonstop during a lifetime, passes through cardiac circuitry, causing the heart to contract and push blood through the chambers and then out into your body.

Heart disease can disrupt this normal electrical and pumping operation. For instance, problems with the electrical system—known as arrhythmias —can make it difficult for the heart to pump blood efficiently. Because of the electrical nature of the heart, it was natural for a curious cardiologist like me to be attracted to energy and electrical concepts that might affect the cardiovascular system in some beneficial way.

In 2001, I was invited to speak at an electromedicine conference in San Diego. That's where I met Clint Ober. He had just completed his second study—how grounding affected cortisol and stress—and he was interested in discussing his research with a cardiologist who had an interest in electromedicine. He looked me up at the conference. We talked awhile, and I was immediately intrigued by his concept. Afterward, we met in his RV and talked in more detail. There was another medical doctor present, as well as a researcher who had developed a cuff to measure blood vessel elasticity. The researcher had his device with him and he used it to test our individual elasticity. You want your arteries to be good and elastic. Rigid, constricted blood vessels are symptomatic of high blood pressure and arterial disease. My reading was good, but Clint's was enviously better. He was about two years older than me, so I was very impressed. I remember thinking how could this guy have a better result than me? Here I was, the big prevention doctor who wrote books and newsletters about healthy lifestyle!

Clint said in his usual soft-spoken voice that he believed the results had to do with the fact that he grounded himself all the time. He slept grounded, and he walked barefoot whenever possible.

Clint also shared with me his frustration with the medical and scientific community that had shown little or no interest in grounding. He was having a hard time getting a foot inside the door of science.

A NEW HEALING FRONTIER

If anything, I felt like a door to a new healing frontier had been pulled open by the most unlikely of individuals. Over my decades of practicing medicine, I had heard countless inspiring talks from the greatest and most honored medical experts. Doctors. Scientists. Professors. Nobel Prize winners. Clint Ober was none of those. He said he was "just" a cable TV guy who had made a discovery he felt could help alleviate suffering. I was impressed by his integrity and intentions. He was somebody with a mission. I felt he was on to something very important and fundamental, with great potential not just for cardiology, but also for the healing community at large. He had just a bare beginning of scientific evidence to back up his observations. Nevertheless, as a cardiologist, it made a lot of sense to me. In addition, my intuition was telling me this was big and exciting and on the mark.

For years, I had been doing a lot of research and writing about antioxidants. In my cardiac practice, I had found that antioxidant nutritional supplements, such as CoQ_{10}, gave a clinically significant healing boost to my patients. I was curious as to whether there was an antioxidant and inflammation connection to Clint's discovery.

Just a year or so before, Harvard researchers had published strong evidence to show that chronic inflammation was a leading cause of arterial disease that chokes off blood, nutrients, and oxygen to the heart and brain, resulting in heart attacks and stroke.

So inflammation and antioxidants were on my mind when I met Clint. I asked him about inflammation. Could grounding reduce inflammation? If it did, grounding might represent a new weapon against heart disease, the No. 1 disease killer in America, and many other common conditions linked to inflammation.

I didn't know the answer. Clint didn't know.

I asked if he could find out.

He said he would. And he did, pretty much on his own at first, and later with the help of a terrific biophysicist, James Oschman.

EARTH/BODY MEDICINE

Clint, with his knowledge of electricity and grounding cable TV systems, now began to exhaustively study physiology and the immune system. He quickly began putting two and two together. Electrical engineers know that the surface of the Earth is pulsating with free electrons. Medical scientists didn't know that, but they did know that the body is electrical in nature, and that free radical molecules attract electrons and snatch them from other molecules, a process at the core of inflammation, tissue destruction, and disease. Clint theorized that if Earthing reduces pain, it must come from reducing or neutralizing the free radicals causing the pain during the inflammatory process. The free electrons must be putting out the fire.

Clint called me one day, excited about having found another important explanation for how grounding was working in the body. It didn't "just" normalize cortisol, improve sleep, and reduce stress, as if those weren't enough. If somebody is in direct contact with the Earth—barefoot or through one of his grounded pads—the free electrons flow into the conductive circuitry of the body and snuff out inflammation. Inflammation causes pain. People with pain who are grounded experience less pain.

For him, the connection was simple.

Get grounded.

Get well.

Get pain relief.

Heal.

People talk about mind/body medicine. I've been practicing that for years. I never heard anybody talk about earth/body medicine before Clint.

To me, this was another landmark finding, a major breakthrough. This was literally electromedicine from the ground up. A secret of the ages right under my feet. For me, the original anti-inflammatory and the ultimate antioxidant had been found.

SLEEPING AND FISHING GROUNDED

After meeting Clint, I had obtained one of his prototype mattress pads and started sleeping grounded. The difference was profound. My wife and I were both able to fall asleep faster. I still use that same pad to this day. I wrote about sleeping grounded in my health newsletter in 2002, and a number of my subscribers obtained a bed pad for themselves. Some took the time to give me feedback afterward and said it had made a difference in their lives.

In time, as I became involved in some of Clint's research projects and heard the feedback from people whose heart functions had improved, the exciting potential of Earthing as a tool against heart disease started to crystallize.

I travel a good deal, giving lectures and attending medical conferences, and sleeping in hotels has always been problematic. Later on, when Clint designed some portable models, we were able to sleep grounded on the road just as we did at home. Now I never leave home without my pad, and I'm always looking for opportunities to walk barefoot.

For years, I used to suffer with flare-ups of psoriasis, a common inflammatory condition of the skin. It would appear on my lower legs and elbows. I had always noticed that whenever I would go bonefishing off the Florida coast—a favorite recreational pursuit of mine—the psoriasis would virtually disappear for weeks afterward. I attributed that to the healing influence of being out in the sun, the vitamin D, the minerals in the saltwater, and time off from the daily stresses of a busy cardiology practice. In bonefishing, you spend hours casting for fish with a fly rod while walking on white sand flats knee-deep in crystal clear water. After meeting Clint, I realized that there was another reason for the improvement of the psoriasis. I was grounded, barefoot in saltwater that is highly conductive. As I was fishing, I was simultaneously giving myself a treatment. Now that I ground myself at night, the psoriasis is virtually gone.

Bob Tolve, an old fishing buddy of mine from Scarsdale, New York, shared an interesting story with me after I told him about Earthing. Bob is sixty-three, my age, and has been in the construction business for many years. When he started out as a young man, he worked for a while with a crew of older carpenters from Norway. He recalled them telling him that if he wanted to last in the business he should do as they do: first thing in the morning go out and walk barefoot on the wet Earth. That would take away the aches and pains of the profession, they said. Bob never forgot the story.

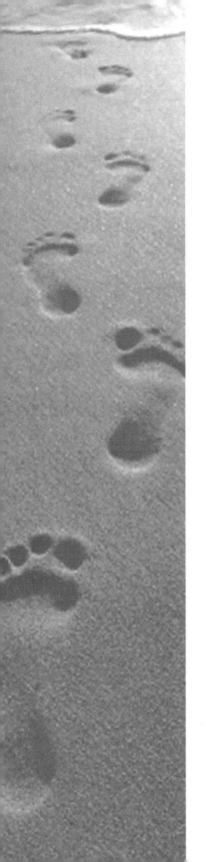

PART THREE

Connecting
with Science

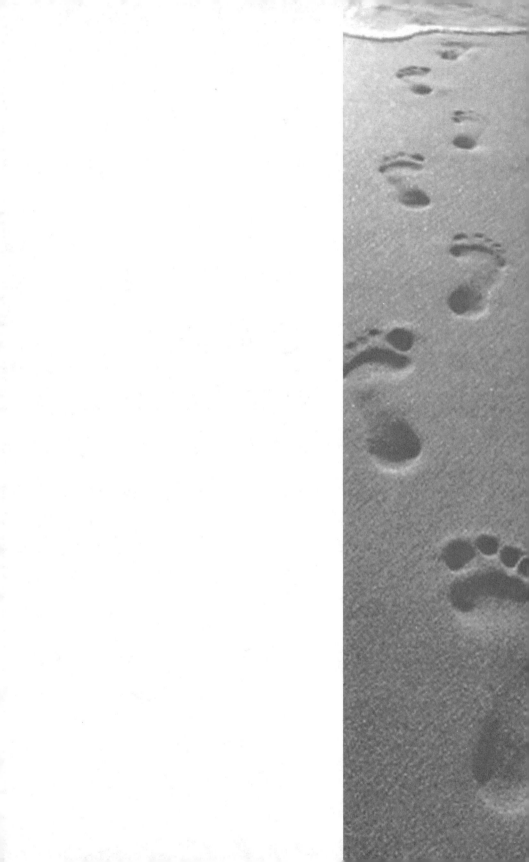

CHAPTER 7

The Original
Anti-Inflammatory

The Earth itself is the original anti-inflammatory. And the planet itself is the biggest electron donor on the planet.

What does this mean to you?

Just imagine a mighty unseen cavalry of free electrons, galloping up through your body from the Earth and mopping up outnumbered forces of inflammatory free radicals. Electron deficiency, created by a lack of grounding, is eliminated and a healing process unfolds.

The inflammation, sickness, and pain in your body are but a manifestation—in large part or small—of an electron deficiency. The remedy is as close as the Earth you live on.

In 2000, Clint Ober was asked by a friend if he would ground an elderly gentleman who was bedridden with advanced rheumatoid arthritis. The man's hands, elbows, and feet were grotesquely misshapen and inflamed. He was wracked with pain and could hardly move and then only very slowly. He was receiving comfort and at-home support from hospice, the national organization that offers services to patients whose life expectancy is six months or less.

Ober said he would come and see what could be done. It took three people to lift the man out of the bed in order to allow a conductive bed pad to be placed on it. The pad was then connected to a ground rod outside.

About ten days later, Ober received a phone call from the man, asking if he could come over again. He said that a squirrel had eaten through the ground wire.

"How do you know that?" Ober wanted to know.

"I went out and saw it had been chewed through," the man said.

Ober was puzzled. How could a bedridden patient be up and about in his yard in a matter of a few days?

"That's what I did," he said. "I went out and saw it."

Astonished, Ober drove up again. He found the man waiting for him, leaning against the front door. He said he was feeling better. And he was right about the wire. It had indeed been chewed up by an animal. Ober replaced it.

After the elderly patient had used the bed pad for a year, Ober learned from his friend that the man was much improved. He was doing household chores, tending to his fireplace, and even carrying firewood into the house from outside. The swelling had gone down. He was stronger, and he moved, talked, and expressed himself with new liveliness. The friend said that the once bedridden man had told him, "I feel I no longer have disease in my body."

The man continued to sleep grounded every night for the next five years until he died.

This remarkable turnaround is nothing more than Earth energy in action. It reveals the largely unknown fact that the ground represents the biggest and best natural antioxidant and anti-inflammatory that exists.

In this chapter, we will describe the healing connection between the Earth and physical inflammation. You'll get an idea how this connection

What Is Inflammation?

Everyone is susceptible to inflammation—from high-performance athletes to non-performance couch potatoes. It's an equal opportunity hit man.

The word "inflammation" comes from the Latin *inflammatio,* meaning to set on fire. Inflammation is the complex biological response of the body to harmful stimuli, such as pathogens, damaged cells, or irritants. It is a protective attempt by the system to remove injurious or threatening agents as well as start the healing process for the affected tissue. In the absence of inflammation, wounds and infections would never heal and progressive destruction of the tissue would compromise survival.

has unlimited potential to reinfuse health and defuse pain among disconnected societies where there is increasing sickness despite all the money poured into medical research and treatments.

But before we get back to the Earth and how it snuffs out inflammation, let's first look at what inflammation is (see the inset on opposite page).

Your immune system protects you against pathogens and facilitates the rebuilding of tissue at sites of injury or surgery. When a problem develops someplace, your body does the equivalent of calling 911. The alarm sounds. White blood cells and other specialized cells rush to the site—the first responders. The white blood cells constantly cruise throughout the tissues of your body, like police patrol cars, ever on the alert for viruses, bacteria, or other alien microorganisms, as well as damaged cells created by trauma or internal irritants. As weapons, some of the cells release a shower of powerful free radicals (called an oxidative burst) that aid in the destruction of invading microorganisms and damaged tissue.

Free radicals have gotten a bad rap, and you will see why in a minute, but in reality they perform an essential service to the body. Simply put, they are electron-hungry molecules (needing one or more electrons to stabilize their molecular structure). You can call them electrophiles—electron lovers. Normally, these free radicals obtain their electrons by stripping them away from pathogens and damaged tissue. This activity kills the bad bugs you want out of your body and breaks down damaged cells for removal. As the remedial work winds down, excess free radicals produced during the immune response are neutralized by antioxidants or free electrons in the body.

This response is triggered whenever you have a disease or an injury. It is called the "inflammatory response." As a result, you may feel the familiar signs and symptoms of inflammation: swelling, redness, heat, and pain, and, depending where the site is, decreased range of motion.

CHRONIC INFLAMMATION = ELECTRON DEFICIENCY

Inflammation comes in two forms: acute or chronic. The acute type takes place as an initial response of the body to harmful stimuli. It involves the mobilization of plasma (the yellow-colored liquid component of blood) and white blood cells from the blood into the injured tissue, as just described. That's okay. You want that to happen.

Then there is chronic (prolonged) inflammation. That you don't want. Chronic inflammation means a progressive shift in the type of activity going on at the site of inflammation. You get simultaneous destruction and healing of the tissue, but a harmful free-radical encroachment into healthy, surrounding territory. The destruction derby continues, and it can seriously harm you.

Free radicals obviously have starring roles in the immune response, but problems arise when the process fails to wind down completely after the job is done. The good guys become bad guys on a rampage, ripping up innocent, healthy cells. Think of security dogs that snag the burglar and then go after their owner. They continue attacking and oxidize healthy tissue. The immune system gears switch into overdrive, sending in more white blood cells that produce more free radicals. This activity is why free radicals have a bad rap and why scientists unanimously agree that free-radical activity is at the basis of chronic disease and the aging process, particularly accelerated aging and limited life span.

We believe that normal inflammation veers out of control because of lost contact with the Earth. People are suffering from an electron deficiency—not enough free electrons on hand to satisfy the lust of rampaging free radicals. They continue to attack the adjacent neighborhood of healthy tissue in an ever-expanding vicious cycle. The nonstop attack mode generates an autoimmune response manifesting as chronic inflammation. The immune system has run amok, attacking its owner—you.

We've simplified the scenario, but this is basically how it works. A destructive process unfolds that can continue silently and indefinitely even for dozens of years and lead to so many intractable modern diseases. Earlier we mentioned the new scientific term for this—inflamm-aging. Now you can see where it comes from.

INFLAMMATION AS A DISEASE-MAKER

The idea that chronic inflammation could be involved in disease began to gain serious attention over twenty-five years ago. At that time, two Australian researchers, Barry Marshall and Robin Warren, reported for the first time that stomach ulcers were not caused by stress or spicy food but by inflammation triggered during bacterial infection. This discovery earned the pair a Nobel Prize.

A subsequent breakthrough occurred in the field of cardiology. Back in the mid-1800s, the famous German pathologist Rudolph Virchow had recognized that injured and inflamed arteries might be a source of heart attacks. His idea failed to gain traction during his time and faded away. Later, during most of the last half of the twentieth century, the cholesterol theory emerged, and since then lowering cholesterol has become a medical obsession and a multi-billion dollar business for pharmaceutical and food manufacturers. However, medical research has shown that half of all heart attacks and strokes occur among people with normal cholesterol levels. So during the 1980s, some cardiologists began to reexamine Virchow's ideas about inflammation.

The breakout came in a series of important studies beginning in 2000. Evidence from a women's study that monitored 28,000 initially healthy postmenopausal women introduced a new cardiovascular risk factor into the spotlight: C-reactive protein (CRP), a biochemical substance measured in the blood that indicates the presence of inflammation. People with the highest level of CRP had five times the risk of developing cardiovascular disease and four times the risk of a heart attack or stroke compared to individuals with the lowest level. CRP, the researchers said, predicted risk in women who had none of the standard risk factors and was the best predictor among twelve risk factors studied, including cholesterol. Harvard cardiologist Paul Ridker, M.D., the lead researcher, said, "We have to think of heart disease as an inflammatory disease, just as we think of rheumatoid arthritis as an inflammatory disease."

Dr. Ridker estimated that approximately 25 percent of Americans have normal to low cholesterol, lulling them into complacency, but at the same time they have elevated CRP they don't know about. This means that millions are currently unaware they have an increased risk for future cardiovascular trouble.

In the arteries, think of low-grade inflammation as a silent, creeping fire that consumes tissue. It leads to the weakening and eventual rupture of arterial plaques that directly trigger heart attacks and stroke. The CRP-inflammation link helps explain why so many heart attack and stroke victims have normal cholesterol levels.

Another example of a common disorder increasingly being seen as inflammation-related is diabetes. In type 1 diabetes, the kind that affects youngsters, the body's immune system attacks the pancreatic cells that make insulin. Insulin is the hormone responsible for controlling the blood sugar level and opening cell "doors" to sugar for use in energy production. Research also suggests that type 2 diabetes, the most common form of the disease and generally occurring in adulthood, begins with insulin resistance. This means that energy production stops responding properly to insulin. The reason for this, researchers believe, is an excess of inflammatory substances released from fatty tissue, particularly in the abdomen. Fat cells, once thought to be merely storage depots for energy and metabolically inert, are now known to be hotbeds of inflammation. This connection helps explain why obesity leads to diabetes. In addition, some studies suggest that eating certain foods may stoke more inflammation in the body and raise the risk of diabetes. They include foods high in sugar and other sweeteners, white flour products, trans fats, polyunsaturated vegetable oils, and processed meats.

It seems that hardly a day goes by without some new study pointing the finger at runaway inflammation as the core of some disease. Inflammatory diseases have become a global epidemic and include some of the most devastating disorders of our times. Table 7-1 lists just a few of them.

Along with the continuing flow of revelations regarding inflammation, researchers have also accumulated much evidence demonstrating that painful conditions are often the result of acute or chronic inflammation. One pain expert has postulated that the origin of all pain is inflammation and the inflammatory response.

Many physicians and researchers wonder what has caused inflammation to become so dangerously commonplace. When asked what causes inflammation in the first place, Harvard's Dr. Ridker said this: "We are witnessing evolutionary biology in action—an adaptive response (inflammation) in the past is now maladaptive in our current modern environment."

The discovery of the relationship of grounding to inflammation suggests that the once adaptive response called inflammation has maybe gone sour because of an electron deficiency from loss of direct contact with the Earth.

TABLE 7-1. CONDITIONS RELATED TO CHRONIC INFLAMMATION

DISEASE	HEALTH EFFECTS
Allergies	Inflammatory messengers stimulate release of histamine, leading to allergic reactions.
Alzheimer's disease	Inflamed brain tissues develop plaque; chronic inflammation kills brain cells.
Amyotrophic lateral sclerosis (ALS)*	Damage to motor neurons causes the body to launch an overzealous inflammatory counterattack, killing the motor neurons.
Anemia	Inflammatory messengers attack red blood cell production.
Arthritis	Chronic inflammation destroys joint cartilage and inhibits the release of lubricating and cushioning fluid in the joints.
Asthma	Inflammation leads to blocking of the bronchial passages.
Autism	Brain inflammation is present in most autistic children.
Cancer	Inflammation contributes to free radicals, tumor growth, and inhibits the body's defense against abnormal cells.
Cardiovascular disease	Inflammation causes thick, unhealthy blood and arterial disease, leading to blockage and plaque and increased risk of dangerous clots in the blood vessels that feed the heart and brain; inflammation also damages heart valves.
Diabetes, types 1 & 2	Type 1 diabetes, inflammation induces the immune system to destroy pancreatic beta cells; type 2 diabetes, fat cells cause the release of inflammatory messengers, leading to insulin resistance.
Fibromyalgia	Inflammatory compounds present in the body at an elevated level.
Common intestinal disorders	Crohn's disease, irritable bowel, diverticulitis, and other intestinal problems involve inflammation that causes pain, interference with digestion and assimilation of nutrients, and damage to the sensitive lining of the digestive tract.
Kidney failure	Inflammation restricts circulation and damages kidney cells that filter blood.
Lupus	Inflammatory compounds spark an autoimmune attack.
Multiple sclerosis	Inflammatory compounds attack the nervous system.
Pain	Activation of pain receptors, transmission and modulation of pain signals, and hypersensitivity of nervous system are all one continuum of inflammation and the inflammatory response.
Pancreatitis	Inflammation induces pancreatic cell injury.
Psoriasis and eczema	Inflammation-based skin disorders.

*ALS is often called Lou Gehrig's disease

ENTER EARTHING: THE MISSING LINK

The land and seas of planet Earth are alive with an endless and constantly replenished supply of electrons. By making direct contact with the surface of the planet, our conductive bodies naturally equalize with the Earth. Figuratively speaking, we refill the electron level in our tank that has become low.

How do we know that the body absorbs those electrons? There are a number of ways we know.

One is common sense. The Earth is negatively charged. It has a virtually infinite supply of free electrons. Anytime you have two conductive objects and they make contact—such as your bare feet and the ground—electrons will flow from the place where they are abundant to the place where there are fewer of them. The electrical potential of the two objects will thus equalize. That's grounding. Similarly, when you stick a ground rod in the Earth, it allows the electrons to flow from the Earth via a wire into an object. It could be a refrigerator, the shielding around a cable TV system, or you. Your body is conductive like the fridge.

Free radicals and electrons constantly interact in high-speed and in highly complex bioelectrochemical exchanges. Many free radicals are regarded in terms of being positively charged molecules, but some can actually be neutral or even negatively charged. These reactive molecules hunger for electrons. The Earth provides the body with a huge influx of electrons and reduces or shuts down the inflammatory destruction attributed to excess free radicals.

If you have a battlefront with electron-seeking free radicals running amok inside your body, guess what's going to happen when you make contact with the Earth?

Big negatively charged Earth overwhelms little electron-hungry free radicals.

Science backs up the common sense. Science tells us that the body is one dynamic conductor of electrical impulses, or in the words of biophysicist James Oschman, "the living matrix." Cells contain an internal framework known as the cytoskeleton that connects all parts of the cell, from the nucleus to the outer membrane. This "scaffolding" includes molecules that conduct energy and information inside each cell and outward to the surrounding environment, and in the opposite direction, from the environment to the innermost parts of the cell and nucleus. Similarly, the surrounding environment, from your head to your toes, contains an extra-cellular network of conductive collagen and other proteins that are "hard-wired" to cell membranes. Thus, the living matrix inside and outside cells provides a body-wide network for antioxidant electrons, a pathway hooking up all parts of the body, including the nervous system and all sensory receptors, with all parts of every cell, including the genome in every cell. This pervasive system has extensions into every nook and cranny of the body and really represents, when you think about it, the largest organ system in the body. It is the "stuff" of all living structures.

When you think of yourself as an "antenna," as the French agronomist Matteo Tavera describes all living things (we discussed his ideas in Chapter 3), you can see how we fit neatly into a universal energy continuum. We, and the stars, are bathed in it.

Michael Jordan and the Living Matrix

Think of the living matrix as a kind of warp-speed communication network inside your body.

Nobel Prize winner Albert Szent-Györgyi, the Hungarian biochemist who first identified vitamin C and was among the first to apply theories of quantum physics to the understanding of cancer, was always a scientist ahead of his time. He laid out the vision of a high-speed communication system in the body—he called it "electronic biology"—back in 1941. He said, "Life is too rapid and subtle to be explained by slow-moving chemical reactions and nerve impulses. The proteins are the stage upon which the drama of life unfolds. The actors can be none other than small and highly mobile units such as electrons and protons."

To illustrate the blazing fast speed of communication within the living matrix, Dr. Oschman uses the analogy of Michael Jordan, one of professional basketball's greatest players. It is the last game and the last seconds of the basketball playoffs. The game is tied, and of course the ball comes to Jordan. In an instant he springs into midair and launches the ball toward the basket. As the buzzer sounds and the game is over, the ball drops through the hoop. Jordan's buzzer-beating shot wins the championship for his team. As the fans go wild, Jordan looks into the TV cameras, smiles, and shrugs his shoulders, as if to say, "Don't ask me how I did that!"

Medical science utilizes the concept of the living matrix in a very practical and helpful way. Doctors use electrophysiological and biomedical instrumentation such as EKGs, EEGs (electroencepthalograms), and EMGs (electromyograms) as diagnostic tools to monitor the electrical activities of the heart, brain, and muscles. These devices follow certain conductive pathways existing between internal organs and the body skin surface, and vice versa. The readings from the interior follow pathways to the skin surface, where they are picked up by electrode patches and led to the measuring devices. Pacemakers, defibrillators, and electroacupuncture demonstrate how this conductivity works in reverse: from the skin to the tissues and organs inside the body.

Electrons are the smallest possible negative charges of electricity. It is well established that negative charges (electrons) are attracted to positive charges. Connecting the body to the Earth automatically enables the conductive tissues of the body's living matrix to become charged with the Earth's free electrons. When this occurs, excess or residual immune response free radicals (which are electron hungry) suddenly have, as the old song goes, the object of their affection—a readily available supply of free electrons to bond with and reduce their oxidative and inflammatory mode. They are neutralized, quenched, satiated, and satisfied. Kind of like giving kids the keys to the ice cream store or opening the blood bank to Dracula.

As a result, the addiction of immune system-produced free radicals to oxidize healthy tissue to obtain their fix of missing electrons naturally disappears. The rampage is naturally inhibited, and with it the underlying mechanism of chronic inflammation and autoimmune disease. The body naturally conducts, and becomes charged with, the Earth's free electrons; that is, it equalizes with and maintains the natural electrical potential of the Earth. The end result, our observations and research indicate, is that the reconnection prevents or reduces chronic inflammation and consistently speeds recovery from exhaustion, acute trauma, and minor injuries. You'll read how that plays out in the very dramatic stories we've collected in Part Four of the book.

Typically, there's a quick reduction in inflammation-related aches and pain. Some acute headaches can vanish within minutes. The intensity of chronic pains often lessens significantly in twenty to forty minutes.

The effect of Earthing on inflammation and pain was dramatically demonstrated in a series of case studies conducted with thermography during 2004 and 2005. Thermography, also known as infrared imaging, is a noninvasive clinical technique that analyzes the skin surface temperatures as a reflection of normal or abnormal human physiology. The technique utilizes sophisticated computerized technology to translate temperature data and produce an image that is then evaluated for signs of possible disease or injury. The procedure has been around for more than thirty years and featured in thousands of medical studies. Among other things, it is widely used to help diagnose breast cancer, diabetes, nervous system and metabolic disorders, injuries, headaches and pain syndromes, neck and back problems, and arterial disease.

William Amalu, D.C., president of the International Academy of Clinical Thermography, performed Earthing studies on twenty patients with a variety of complaints, including chronic myofascial pain syndrome, muscular strains, ligamentous sprains, peripheral neuropathies, carpal tunnel syndrome, inflammatory joint conditions, Lyme's disease, and chronic sinusitis. The subjects were either grounded with conductive electrode patches in his office or slept on grounded bed pads at home. The results showed, through dramatic pictures, a major and rapid impact on inflammation and pain. A picture is worth a thousand words, so please refer to the color images (Plates 1–4) on pages 81–84 showing some of these changes.

Some patients experienced improvement in just one session. Within two to four weeks (of two to three half-hour treatments weekly), up to 80 percent improvement occurred in the cases that were followed up (60 percent of cases were followed). With ongoing grounding over weeks and months, the patients continued to get relief, feel better, and in some cases, their symptoms vanished altogether.

"The moment your foot touches the Earth, or you connect to the Earth through a wire, your physiology changes," James Oschman says. "An immediate normalization begins. And an anti-inflammatory switch is turned on. People stay inflamed because they never connect with the Earth, the source of free electrons, which can neutralize the free radicals in the body that cause disease and cellular destruction."

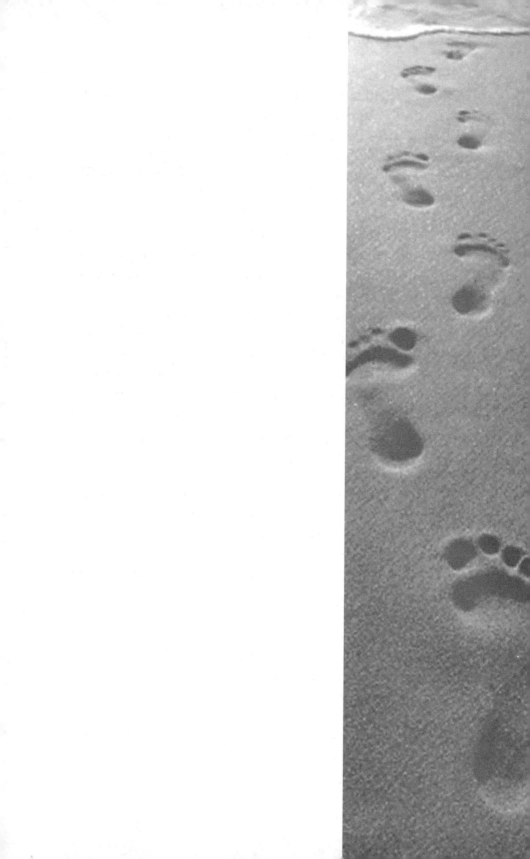

CHAPTER 8

Connecting
the Dots

Gaétan Chevalier is a hard-nosed Southern California biophysicist and electrophysiologist, a scientist specializing in the body's electrical "wiring." In the summer of 2008, he conducted a study to investigate the impact of Earthing on a variety of physiological functions in the body. During preliminary work to test the design of the study, he invited a friend—a retired probation officer—to the laboratory to act as a "guinea pig." The subjects in the experiment were going to be grounded while sitting in a comfortable reclining chair, similar to one you may have in your living room. The friend sat down in the chair, and Clint Ober started chatting with him.

"A few minutes into the conversation, my friend mentioned that he had painful arthritis in his hands, something I hadn't known about," recalled Dr. Chevalier. "Clint then asked him to describe his current level of pain on a scale of 0 to 10, with 10 being unbearable pain.

"My friend described his level as 8 in the left and 9 in the right.

"Clint then placed an electrode patch on the palm of each hand and snapped on a wire connected to an outside ground rod. We continued to talk. After about a half hour, Clint asked my friend about the pain level now.

"A look of surprise came over my friend's face. He suddenly became aware that his pain level had dropped way down. He answered 2 on the left and 3 on the right, and then said, 'I have not experienced so little pain in my hands for a long time. This is amazing.'"

Dr. Chevalier described a similar experience with one of his yoga instructors. She had severe arthritis in the thumbs, and doing something

71

as simple as picking up an object—a cup, for instance—would often produce shooting pain up into the arm so bad that she dropped the object.

"She came to the laboratory and we grounded her for a half hour," he said. "When she left, she told us she didn't feel any pain. I see her every week at yoga class, and after several months she said that the pain in the thumbs never came back. She now walks on the beach for at least a half-hour every day and also sleeps grounded."

Observations like these have been commonplace right from the start of the pursuit of scientific validation for Earthing. The positive results in the early studies prompted deeper and more sophisticated investigations about how grounding affects the body and its complicated inner machinery. Now, a decade after the first experiment, ongoing research has started to put together the pieces of this amazing story into a multifaceted hypothesis with great implications for human health. In this chapter, we will present some of the most revealing and important findings to date.

THE NUTS AND BOLTS OF EARTHING

A study published in 2005 by electrical engineer Roger Applewhite confirmed two highly significant facts:

1. Electrons move from the Earth to the body and vice versa when the body is grounded. This effect is sufficient to maintain the body at the same electrical potential as the Earth.

2. Grounding powerfully reduces alternating current (AC) voltages induced on the body by ambient electromagnetic fields (EMFs).

It is hard to avoid electro-technical language to describe this important study that demonstrates some basic physics behind Earthing, and specifically that the human body is a natural conductor of the Earth's vibrant surface energy. We will do our best to keep things simple.

Mr. Applewhite is an expert in the design of electrostatic discharge systems for high-tech and electronic industries. His study, published in the journal *European Biology and Bioelectromagnetics,* involved a series of electrical measurements on the body of an individual grounded and ungrounded. Grounding was achieved by attaching conductive electrode patches to various places on the anatomy or by lying on a conductive bed sheet.

A voltage drop across an in-line resistor, measured with an oscilloscope, provided ample evidence of an exchange of electrons between the Earth and the body during grounding.

The electric potential (in volts) generated on the body by the EMFs at 60 Hz was recorded on both the ungrounded and grounded body using a specially designed high-impedance measurement system. Earthing, either with the patches or the bed sheet, reduced the immediate environmental electric potential by a factor of at least 70. Figure 8-1 below shows this knockdown effect graphically.

Thus, in one study, the Earth connection was shown to serve as a "source" of beneficial electrons and, at the same time, as a "shield" preventing environmental electric fields from creating disruptive electric potentials on the body.

EARTHING TRUMPS EMFS

In recent years, there has been much discussion in scientific circles and in the media about the possible health effects from exposure to man-made EMFs. Because of widespread interest in this issue, we would like to take a moment and attempt to shed additional light on the subject in relation to grounding.

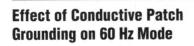

Effect of Conductive Patch Grounding on 60 Hz Mode

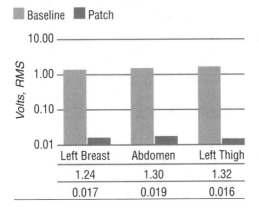

	Left Breast	Abdomen	Left Thigh
	1.24	1.30	1.32
	0.017	0.019	0.016

Figure 8-1.
The graph shows the huge difference in environmental electric field potential measured on the body at three sites—at baseline, that is, before grounding, and during grounding.

All of us live immersed in an unseen sea of human-generated EMFs. They are everywhere—in our houses, workplaces, and outdoors—primarily produced by the electrical power grid. In North America, the grid produces EMFs vibrating at 60 Hz. Existing wires inside the walls produce EMFs even when appliances are not connected. The potential for interference in our bodies varies from person to person and in different locations, depending on the intensity of the fields. Within an ungrounded body, electrons and other charged particles react with the EMFs present in the immediate environment producing unnatural perturbations. When a person is grounded, the body is shielded from these perturbations by the Earth's electrons.

Some individuals are ultrasensitive and can be severely affected. This "electrical hypersensitivity" cannot be explained by any known mechanisms, as the threshold for known interactions is at least fifty times higher than actual exposure levels. Nevertheless, we believe that hypersensitivity is a real phenomenon that may be related to stress and the disconnect with the Earth. In Chapter 12, you will read a dramatic story of debilitating electrical hypersensitivity. To us, the ungrounded body "floats" in a tempest of random environmental energies and operates unstably, like a leaf in the wind.

The Applewhite study we just described showed that when the body is directly connected to the Earth, it is essentially shielded from electropollution. This finding confirms what is generally accepted in basic physics (see the inset "The Umbrella Effect of Earthing" on pages 76–77) and also substantiates what we learned while doing the cortisol study described in Chapter 5. In that experiment, twelve subjects were grounded to the Earth during sleep. Their electrical field–induced body voltage, from exposure to common electrical wiring and cords near their beds, was measured before and after grounding.

What most people don't realize is that if you sleep with a lamp, clock, or radio next to your bed, the electric field from the wires will extend out to your body, even if the appliances are turned off. As measured by a voltmeter, in the bedrooms of the study subjects there was an average of about 3.3 volts pregrounding. The level was significantly reduced, averaging 0.007 volts, when subjects slept on the grounded bed pads. The stark differences, and protective effect of grounding, are summarized in Table 8-1.

TABLE 8-1. ELECTRICAL FIELD-INDUCED VOLTAGE CREATED ON SUBJECTS' BODIES WHILE LYING IN THEIR OWN BEDS		
SUBJECTS	VOLTS BEFORE GROUNDING	VOLTS AFTER GROUNDING
1	3.94	0.003
2	1.47	0.001
3	2.70	0.004
4	1.20	0.002
5	2.70	0.005
6	1.67	0.005
7	5.95	0.008
8	3.94	0.008
9	3.75	0.010
10	2.30	0.009
11	5.98	0.020
12	3.64	0.006
AVG	3.27	0.007

Our conclusion is further supported by the findings of a team of researchers from the Imperial College in London and the University of Washington's Department of Environmental and Occupational Health Sciences. In a 2007 report, they said that measurements in an office setting showed that the electrical energies people are exposed to indoors for large periods of time escalate the risk of infection, stress, and degenerative diseases, and reduce oxygen uptake and activity levels. "The nature of the electromagnetic environments that most humans are now regularly exposed to has changed dramatically over the past century and often bears little resemblance to those created in Nature," they wrote. "In particular, the increased masking/shielding of individuals from beneficial types of natural electromagnetic phenomena, the presence of synthetic materials that can gain strong charge and increase exposures to inappropriate electric field levels and polarities have greatly altered the electromagnetic nature of the microenvironments many individuals usually occupy."

The Umbrella Effect of Earthing

The Applewhite study showed the protective effect of Earthing against environmental electrical fields. Another way to think of this is as an umbrella effect.

Let us look for a moment at the electrical properties of the Earth's surface and the way the Earth's energy influences our biology. In his classic *Lectures on Physics* from the early 1960s, Nobel Prize physicist Richard Feynman describes the Earth's subtle energies. The surface, as we have seen, has an abundance of electrons, which give it a negative electrical charge. If you are standing outside on a clear day, wearing shoes or standing on an insulating surface (like a wood or vinyl floor), there is an electrical charge of some 350 volts between the Earth and the top of your head (see drawing, left) if you are 5 feet 9 inches (1.75 m) tall. Keep in mind it is about zero volts at ground level.

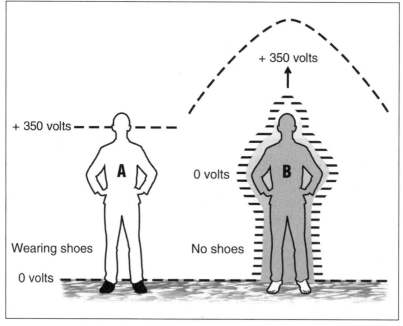

Figure 8-2. The umbrella effect of Earthing.

You might ask, "If there really is a voltage difference of 350 volts from head to toe why don't I get a shock when I go outside?"

The answer is that air is a relatively poor conductor and has virtually no electrical current flow. If you are standing outside in your bare feet (see drawing, right), you are Earthed; your whole body is in electrical contact with the Earth's surface. Your body is a relatively good conductor. Your skin and the Earth's surface make a continuous charged surface with the same electrical potential.

Also notice in the drawing on the right that the charged area is pushed up and away from your head if you are grounded. Any object in direct contact with the Earth—a person, a dog, a tree—creates this shielding effect. The object is essentially residing within the protective umbrella of Earth's natural electric field. This protective phenomenon also occurs inside your house or office, if you are connected to the Earth with an Earthing device like a bed pad.

One of the factors contributing to the potential consequences of electropollution, they said, was the "failure to appropriately ground conductive objects (including humans)."

EARTHING PRODUCES UNIQUE ELECTRICAL FUNCTION IN BRAIN AND MUSCLES

In 2003, electrophysiologists Gaétan Chevalier and Kazuhito Mori at the California Institute for Human Science investigated the impact of Earthing on nervous system function. Fifty-eight healthy adults participated in the randomized, double-blind experiment involving a series of sophisticated brain and muscle measurements. In individual sessions, a conductive adhesive electrode patch was placed on the sole of each participant's foot while seated comfortably in a recliner. The patches were connected to a wire leading outside through a door. Half the participants were actually grounded, that is, the wire was connected to a ground rod, thus replicating the act of sitting or standing barefoot outside. The other participants were not grounded. They were similarly patched, but the wires were not connected outside to the rod. Individuals were then monitored, first for a half-hour pretest baseline period and then immediately for another half hour when they were either grounded or "sham" grounded.

The sham group served as what researchers refer to as "controls." The purpose was to make sure the documented effects were real and not just due to people sitting and relaxing in a comfortable chair. The randomized experiment was double-blind, meaning that neither the participants nor the researchers knew which group was assigned to real or sham grounding. Blinded research is an important tool in many fields of research. Only after the data from the experiment have been recorded do the researchers learn who is who, enabling them to then analyze and compare the results.

EEGs record the electrical signals from your brain as measured on the scalp. Abnormal results may indicate the presence of epilepsy and seizures. EMGs detect the electrical voltage generated by muscle cells. In this study, EMG electrodes were placed on the big shoulder muscles on each side of the neck—the trapezius muscles, so named because of their diamond shape.

The EEG and EMG readings showed that grounding significantly influences the electrical activity of the brain and muscles, even within a mere half hour. In fact, dramatic changes were recorded almost instantly (within two seconds) of Earthing.

In the brain, there was an overall decrease in activity at all frequencies, with a crisp change showing on the left side—the one associated with thinking. Thus, Earthing appears to calm down the busy mind.

As far as the muscles were concerned, Earthing produced two intriguing results:

1. Participants with a high level of tension showed a decrease in muscle tension (on both sides). Individuals with little or no muscle tension showed an increase in tension. The result suggests that grounding reestablishes a normal level of tension. The finding paralleled the effect of the earlier cortisol study in which a normalization of the stress-related cortisol level was seen.

2. The grounded subjects—but not the ungrounded ones—showed large and very slow oscillations (between twenty and forty seconds per oscillation, depending on the individual). This type of oscillation has never been seen before in physiology research.

Keep in mind that the body operates electrically, including your muscles. Nerve impulses instruct muscle fibers to contract. The contractions naturally generate electricity and small mechanical vibrations, both of which produce fluctuating frequencies of electrical potential at the surface of the skin. This is the electric "noise" that EMG measures. An oscillation (a slow vibration) means that the contractions generate electricity in a more rhythmic pattern. An analogy would be to compare people walking randomly in a crowd without any particular order versus a military unit marching in unison. The unit is more coherent than a random crowd. The influence of Earthing on muscles suggests more orderly and efficient activity.

The results of this study call for an experiment designed to determine whether greater electrical coherence translates to muscles being able to work longer and harder without fatigue. In Chapter 14, we present examples of grounded athletes describing enhanced performance. The implications for improved muscle function go far beyond athletes to the possibility that elderly individuals, at a time of life when they normally lose muscle strength, may achieve longer muscle "mileage" as a consequence of incorporating Earthing into their lifestyles. We believe the findings may represent a normal mode of muscle function not hitherto observed simply because no studies before have involved grounded subjects! Such precedence aside, the overall results provided additional proof of reduced stress and tension levels, and a shift in nervous system balance from a stress-stimulated sympathetic mode to a calmer parasympathetic mode. The study was published in a 2006 issue of the journal *European Biology and Bioelectromagnetics*.

EARTHING "ENERGIZES" MAJOR ACUPUNCTURE CHANNELS

When we walk barefooted, the front part of the sole (closest to the ball of the foot) comes in connection with the Earth. According to traditional Chinese medicine, this area includes a major acupuncture point known as kidney 1 (K1). The point is a major entryway for the absorption of Earth Qi—the Earth's energy—and connects farther up in the body with the urinary bladder (UB) meridian. UB is an energy channel that reaches many of the most important organs and parts of the body, including the liver, diaphragm, heart, lungs, and brain, as well as a central meridian junction point in the back.

In a second phase of the electrophysiology study described a moment ago, Drs. Chevalier and Mori took the same fifty-eight participants and monitored them for nearly a half hour while ungrounded and then another half hour while grounded. Electrode patches were placed at the K1 point, thus simulating walking barefooted on the ground. (See Figure 8-3.)

The researchers wired up each participant and took detailed electrical measurements at more than two dozen meridian points on the body. They found that grounding generated readings indicative of reduced inflammation and energized internal organs. The results further supported earlier findings showing reduction of internal organ tension and inflammation, as well as increased parasympathetic activity in the nervous system.

This study suggests that "expressways" of electron transfer from the Earth through the body run through highly conductive water-control meridians (involving the kidneys and bladder) and the K1-UB "mainline" connecting many parts and organs of the body. The report was published in the journal *Subtle Energy and Energy Medicine* in 2007.

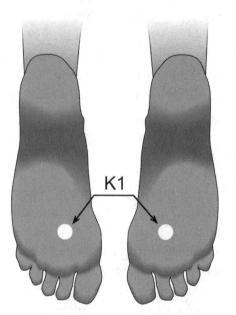

Figure 8-3.
K1 acupuncture point.

THERMAL & PHOTOGRAPHIC IMAGES
OF THE EFFECTS OF EARTHING

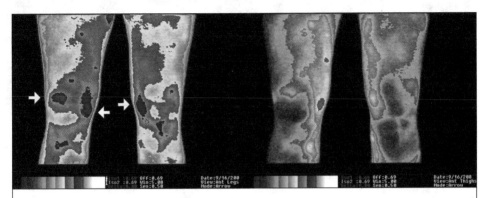

Plate 1. Inflammation as seen through infrared imaging. Thermal imaging cameras record tiny changes in the temperature of the skin to create a color-coded image map. Because tissue damage causes increased heat, abnormally hot areas indicate inflammation. The infrared photos shown here were taken only thirty minutes apart—before (left) and after grounding (right). They illustrate a rapid resolution of inflammation and help explain the impact of Earthing on chronic pain, stiffness, and a variety of symptoms.

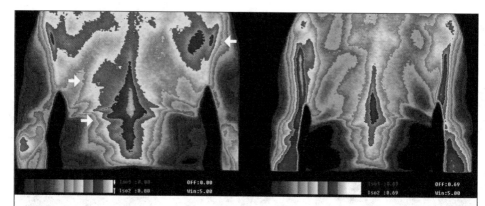

Plate 2. The patient here was an eighty-five-year-old male who complained of intense, left lower back pain and right shoulder pain that interfered with sleep, and waking stiff and sore. Prolonged medical treatment had achieved poor results. After two nights of sleeping grounded, he reported 50 percent less pain and 75 percent less stiffness and soreness when walking. Image (left) shows intense areas of inflammation and pain, denoted by arrows. Image (right), taken after the second night, shows a return to normal thermal symmetry. After four weeks, the patient reported total resolution of back and shoulder pain with only occasional mild stiffness. "I have my life back," he said.

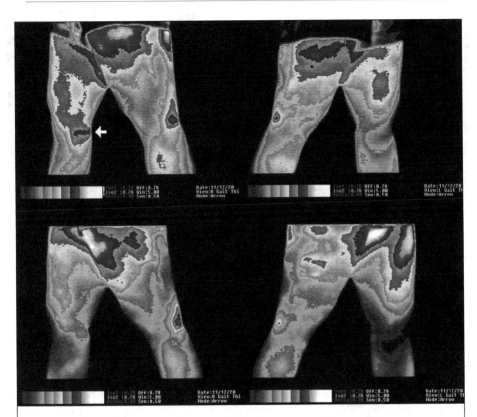

Plate 3. Infrared images are those of a thirty-three-year-old woman who had a gymnastics injury at age fifteen. The patient had a long history of chronic right knee pain, swelling, and instability and was unable to stand for long periods. Simple actions, such as driving, increased the symptoms. She needed to sleep with a pillow between her knees to decrease the pain. On-and-off medical treatment and physical therapy over the years provided minimal relief. Images (top) were taken in walking position to show the inside of both knees. The arrow points to exact location of patient's pain and shows significant inflammation. Images (bottom) were taken thirty minutes after being grounded with an electrode patch. The patient reported a mild reduction in pain. Note the significant reduction of inflammation in the knee area. After six days of grounding, she reported a 50 percent reduction in pain and said that she could now stand for longer periods without pain and no longer needed a pillow between her legs when she slept. After four weeks of treatment, she felt good enough to play soccer and for the first time in fifteen years felt no instability and little pain. By twelve weeks, she said her pain had diminished by nearly 90 percent and she had no swelling. For the first time in many years, she was able to waterski. Six months after initial treatment, she completed running a half-marathon.

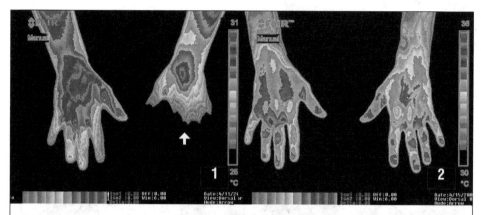

Plate 4. This set of infrared images shows the response to Earthing of a forty-nine-year-old woman with chronic neck and upper back pain that interfered with sleep and daily functioning. She also complained of leg achiness and restless legs during sleep and woke up stiff and sore. Previous medical and alternative treatments had not proven effective. After four nights of sleeping grounded, she reported the following: nearly 70 percent less pain; nearly 30 percent reduction in disturbed sleep; more than 40 percent reduction of sleep-related disturbance in daytime activities; 75 percent less achy and restless legs during sleep; and 80 percent reduction in morning stiffness and soreness. After a six-week follow-up, she reported steady improvements. Image 1 shows her hands prior to grounding. Notice the coolness and poor circulation in the fingers. The arrow points to one hand with temperature so low that the fingers are at the same temperature as the room and cannot be registered (referred to as "thermal amputation"). Image 2 shows how Earthing "warmed up" her hands.

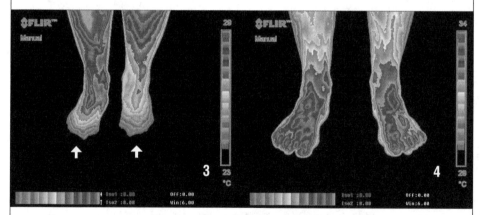

Image 3 shows the lower extremities before Earthing. Arrows point to areas of poor circulation. The low temperature of the toes is similar to the ambient temperature and could not be registered. Image 4, taken after four nights of sleeping grounded, demonstrates significantly improved circulation and a "warming up" of the feet.

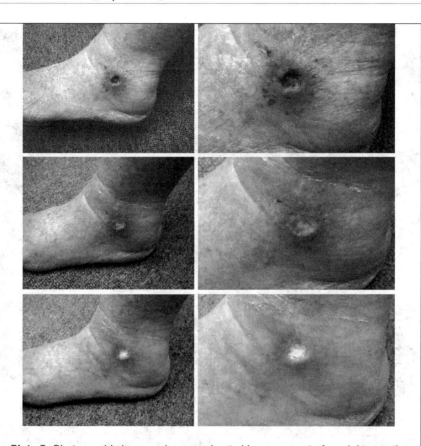

Plate 5. Photographic images show accelerated improvement of an eight-month-old nonhealing open wound suffered by an eighty-four-year-old diabetic woman. Right column pictures are close-ups of the photos to the left. The top row shows the open wound and a pale-gray hue to the skin. Middle row photos, taken after one week, show a marked level of healing and improvement in circulation, as indicated by the skin color. The bottom row, taken after two weeks, shows the wound healed over and the skin color looking dramatically healthier. Treatment consisted of a daily thirty-minute grounding session with an electrode patch while seated comfortably. The cause of the wound adjacent to the left ankle was a poorly fitted boot. A few hours after wearing the boot, a blister formed, and then developed into a resistant open wound. The patient had undergone various treatments at a specialized wound center with no results. Vascular imaging of her lower extremities revealed poor circulation. When first seen, she had a mild limp and was in pain. After an initial thirty minutes of exposure to grounding, the patient reported a noticeable decrease in pain. After one week of daily grounding, she said her pain level was about 80 percent less. At that time, she showed no evidence of a limp. At the end of two weeks, she said she was completely pain-free.

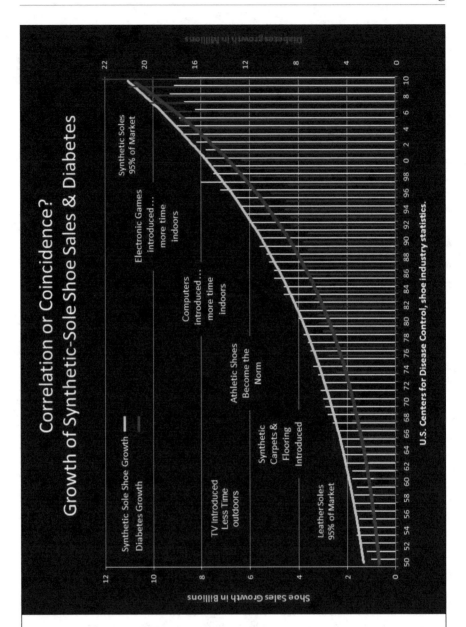

Plate 6. Chart shows a similar curve growth in the incidence of type 2 diabetes and sales of synthetic-sole shoes in the U.S. since the 1950s. At that time, 95 percent of shoes were made with leather soles, many of which were conductive. Currently, 95 percent of shoes have synthetic, nonconductive soles. A similar pattern exists for other health conditions as well.

MORE EFFICIENT CARDIOVASCULAR, RESPIRATORY, NERVOUS SYSTEM FUNCTION

Reconnecting yourself to the Earth may not produce the same effect as jump-starting a dead battery, but it does work surprisingly fast to reenergize fatigued bodies and reduce pain. Earthing usually generates a healing response that people feel after twenty to thirty minutes. Pain reduction can occur much faster.

In an attempt to clock the speed of Earthing, so to speak, a study was organized by Dr. Chevalier to measure different physiological values before, during, and after a forty-minute grounding session. Twenty-seven healthy men and women, ages eighteen to eighty, were used in the experiment. They were grounded with electrode patches applied to the soles of their feet and the palms of their hands. For comparison, measurements were also taken during a similar length session of sham grounding.

Actual grounding produced the following results:

- An immediate reduction (within a few seconds) of skin conductance, indicating rapid activation of the calming-mode parasympathetic nervous system. Skin conductance is a widely accepted measure of nervous system function. This result strengthens our understanding about stress reduction and improved sleep from grounding.

- An increased respiration rate and stabilization of blood oxygenation, as well as a slight rise in heart rate. These changes occurred about twenty minutes after grounding commenced and may suggest the start of a healing response necessitating an increase in oxygen. Signs of more efficient oxygen consumption during grounding continued, as was documented, for at least ten minutes after the cessation of grounding. This fascinating observation links Earthing and a healing response to metabolic activity. We hypothesize that this metabolic activity increase is the source of the healing response and that metabolic activity increases most where the body needs more repair, such as a site of injury or acute inflammation. Interestingly, immediately after ungrounding, blood oxygenation became erratic and respiration rate became even slightly higher. The reaction suggests that the body does not like being "unplugged" from the Earth.

The study, published in 2010 in the *Journal of Alternative and Complementary Medicine,* also showed that the more optimum measurements registered during forty minutes of Earthing shift back—in about ten to twenty minutes—to pregrounding levels after the body is unplugged from the Earth.

POWER HEALING FROM TRAUMA: LESS INFLAMMATION, FASTER RECOVERY

You have undoubtedly experienced delayed onset muscle soreness after engaging in more physical activity than your body was used to. In the fitness and athletic world, this form of misery is called DOMS for short and is a well-known consequence of excessive, unfamiliar, or intensive exercise movements. Plain and simple: overdoing it.

There is no known treatment that reduces the recovery time frame, but massage, hydrotherapy, and acupuncture have a reputation for reducing the pain. DOMS involves acute inflammation in the overtaxed muscles and develops in twenty-four to forty-eight hours. It can persist for well over ninety-six hours.

A study was set up using DOMS as a model to test the impact of Earthing on acute inflammation. Eight healthy males, ages twenty to twenty-three, were put through a similar routine of toe raises while carrying a barbell on their shoulders equal to a third of their body weight. The intense exercise was designed to create tissue injury and pronounced muscle soreness in the calves. In the experiment, each participant was exercised individually on a Monday morning and then monitored for the rest of the week while following a similar eating, sleeping, and living schedule in a hotel. For comparison, the group was divided in half. The men were either actually grounded or sham-grounded throughout the entire week—day and night.

The participants were objectively analyzed in a variety of ways, including through blood draw, MRI, and MRS (magnetic resonance spectroscopy) of the injured tissue. They were also tested daily for pain tolerance at the site of soreness—the calves. A blood pressure cuff was placed around their right gastrocnemius muscle (the big muscle at the back of the lower leg) and slowly inflated until the point of acute discomfort.

The participants also provided subjective responses related to sleep, mood, and muscle soreness.

When inflammation occurs, white blood cells scurry into action. Their numbers increase. Among the ungrounded men, there was an expected, dramatic increase in white blood cells at the stage when DOMS is known to reach its peak and greater perception of pain (see Figure 8-4 on the following page). This result indicates a typical heightened inflammatory response. By comparison, the grounded group experienced a slight decrease in the white blood cell response, indicating almost no inflammation and, for the first time ever documented, a shorter recovery time. At twenty-four, forty-eight, and seventy-two hours after exercise, the white blood count differences between the two groups were 10, 17, and 18 percent.

The researchers looked at a total of forty-eight well-established markers of acute inflammation, DOMS, and pain. In thirty of these markers, a consistent pattern of differences emerged during the testing period.

The study, also published in 2010 in the *Journal of Alternative and Complementary Medicine,* was conducted under the supervision of Dick Brown, Ph.D., a well-known Oregon exercise physiologist and trainer of elite athletes.

"One big thing was the significant difference in the pain that these people felt," commented Dr. Brown. "The men who were grounded not only had a subjective feeling of less pain, but they could also take more pressure applied to their calves with the blood pressure cuffs. Their calves seemed to be less sore.

"Another big thing was the significant differences in the white blood cells and certain compounds in the body. These outcomes clearly invite more investigation, which we plan with a larger subject population.

"I now tell the athletes I train to make every effort to ground themselves. They willingly do so because they have a sense that something is working. They say they have less pain, and that allows them to train more consistently and recover faster. That's a big deal because consistent training is so important to success.

"I personally experienced the benefit of grounding when I had a right knee replacement in 2009. I needed it after years of being physically active at a fairly high level. This is my second knee replacement surgery. The first

Nighttime Pain Scale

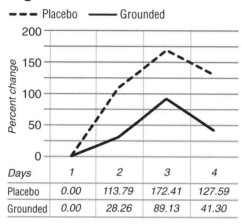

— — Placebo ——— Grounded

Days	1	2	3	4
Placebo	0.00	113.79	172.41	127.59
Grounded	0.00	28.26	89.13	41.30

White Blood Cells

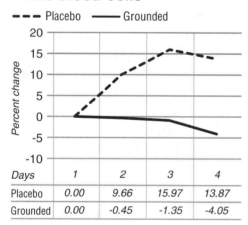

— — Placebo ——— Grounded

Days	1	2	3	4
Placebo	0.00	9.66	15.97	13.87
Grounded	0.00	-0.45	-1.35	-4.05

Figure 8-4.
Delayed muscle onset soreness study.

Ungrounded subjects consistently, at every measurement taken, expressed the perception of greater pain. The difference was on average, 85 percent higher for each day (top graph). Related to this finding was evidence of a subdued white blood cell response, indicating an Earthed body experiences less inflammation (bottom graph).

was ten years ago. Subjectively, I felt I was improving a little bit faster. But five weeks after the operation, when I went to the surgeon for a checkup, he looked at my leg and looked at my movement and said, 'At five weeks, you are where most people are at three months.' He was speaking in terms of movement, wound healing, and swelling. I obviously attribute that partly to my knowledge of rehabbing, but the grounding certainly didn't hurt, and I honestly believe it helped. It had a positive effect.

"I sleep grounded, and I also use grounded electrode patches locally. Before surgery, I noticed that when I put the patches on the area of the knee that was hurting, it definitely reduced the pain compared to when I didn't have the patches on. I needed surgery for about a year but kept putting it off because I had things to do. And so at night, my leg got really painful. So I slept on the grounded sheet and slept better, and further knocked the pain down with the patches."

The careful process of scientific experimentation in the Brown study shows that inflammation is reduced and documents why Earthing has caught on big time in the sports world, where living with inflammation and injury is a way of life. Simply put: the body is different—and heals much faster—when connected to the Earth. Earthing = Power Healing.

LESS RISK OF METABOLIC SYNDROME?

In 2010, Earthing was tested on rodents in a laboratory setting. The unpublished results revealed significant improvements in several bio-chemical factors associated with metabolic syndrome in humans, a wide-spread precursor to obesity, diabetes, and cardiovascular disease.

In the experiment, two healthy groups of thirty rats each were used. One group was housed in cages fitted with grounded mats. The other group, the control animals, lived in similar but ungrounded cages. Blood samples were taken every month for six months and analyzed. Continued grounding resulted in progressive improvements.

The substances monitored were alkaline phosphatase (an enzyme), triglycerides, blood sugar, and C-reactive protein (a widely used indicator of chronic inflammation discussed in the previous chapter). The values of these substances were considerably lower in grounded animals, suggesting less risk for metabolic syndrome. Just as in the DOMS study, there were also fewer white blood cells measured.

The results tie in neatly with the increase in metabolic activity documented in the earlier experiment with human subjects where a relationship between Earthing and a more efficient cardiovascular, respiratory, and nervous system function was observed. It makes sense that an increase in metabolic activity results in a lower risk of developing metabolic syndrome.

The experiment, along with other observations over the years, permit the suggestion—if nothing more at this time—that living in an ungrounded state may be another important cause of metabolic syndrome. One has only to look at today's youth, who generally consume large amounts of inferior quality convenience food and drinks high in sweeteners and

Earthing and Weight Loss? Maybe!

Abdominal obesity is one of the important factors characterizing metabolic syndrome. While such obesity was not measured during the rat study above, the animals were weighed in at the first pretest day and then again at each monthly blood collection time. The random difference in average weight between the two groups of "middle-aged" female rats at the beginning of the study was only 1.2 percent (the ungrounded rodents happened to be insignificantly heavier at the start than the grounded animals) and then grew steadily each month to reach 3.7 percent after six months.

What the numbers mean is that the ungrounded group added an extra 2.6 percent in weight after six months. Both groups were fed the same type and quantity of food. While the difference seems like a trifling amount, it translates to an extra five pounds for a person weighing 200 pounds. At that rate, the difference in weight could grow even larger over a lifetime.

The results, along with the biochemical differences cited in the study, suggest that the grounded rats function at a higher metabolic efficiency than ungrounded animals.

Do these results infer that Earthing can generate weight loss in humans? We can't say. The prospect is certainly tantalizing. Imagine losing weight without doing anything. A dieter's dream.

calories, who are increasingly sedentary, and who wear insulated running shoes from morning to night. For young people as well as for adults, the unholy trinity for metabolic syndrome, and the serious disorders it gives rise to, may thus be poor diet, lack of exercise, and lack of grounding. It is something to think about.

Metabolic syndrome is characterized by a group of metabolic risks that include the following:

- Excessive fat tissue in and around the abdomen.

- Blood fat disorders—high triglycerides, low "healthy" HDL cholesterol, and high "harmful" LDL cholesterol—that contribute to plaque build-ups in arterial walls.

- Elevated blood pressure.

- Insulin resistance or glucose intolerance—conditions that interfere with the body's ability to properly use insulin or blood sugar.

- A tendency to form clots in the blood.

- A pro-inflammatory state in the body, that is, the presence of chemical substances associated with inflammation (such as elevated CRP).

EARTHING STRONGLY INFLUENCES PHYSIOLOGY

In 2010, we were pleased to learn about the work of two Polish doctors who had conducted a series of experiments to determine whether the Earth's natural electric charge influences the regulation of human physiological processes. The physicians are cardiologist Karol Sokal and his neurosurgeon son Pawel. Their research, just as ours, revealed promising and intriguing results and was published in a 2011 issue of the *Journal of Alternative and Complementary Medicine.*

The Sokals set up double-blind experiments with groups ranging from twelve to eighty-four subjects, who followed similar physical activity, diet, and fluid intake during the trial periods. Grounding was achieved with a copper plate (30 mm x 80 mm) placed on the lower part of the leg, attached with a strip so that it would not come off during the night. The plate was connected by a conductive wire to a larger plate (60 mm x 250 mm), which was placed in contact with the Earth outside.

In one experiment with subjects, grounding during one single night of sleep resulted in statistically significant changes in concentrations of minerals and electrolytes in the blood serum: iron, ionized calcium, inorganic phosphorus, sodium, potassium, and magnesium. Renal excretion of both calcium and phosphorus was reduced significantly. The observed reductions in blood and urinary calcium and phosphorus directly relate to osteoporosis. The results suggest that even one night's Earthing exposure reduces primary indicators of osteoporosis.

In another experiment, Earthing continually during rest and physical activity over a seventy-two-hour period decreased fasting glucose among patients with non-insulin-dependent diabetes. Patients had been well controlled with an antidiabetic drug for about six months but at the time of the study were having unsatisfactory blood sugar control despite the medication plus dietary and exercise advice.

In a third experiment, blood samples were drawn from six male and six female adults with no history of thyroid disease. A single night of grounding produced a significant decrease of free triiodothyronine, and an increase of free thyroxine and thyroid-stimulating hormone. The meaning of these results is unclear but suggests an Earthing influence on thyroid metabolism. Interestingly, we have observed that many individuals on thyroid medication reported symptoms of hyperthyroidism (overactive thyroid), such as heart palpitations, after starting grounding. Such symptoms typically vanish after medication is adjusted downward under medical supervision. Through a series of feedback regulations, thyroid hormones affect almost every physiological process in the body, including growth and development, metabolism, body temperature, and heart rate. Clearly, further study of Earthing effects on thyroid function is needed.

In another experiment, the effect of grounding on the classic immune response following vaccination was examined. Earthing accelerated an immune response, as demonstrated by increases in gamma-globulin concentration (antibodies that help the immune system fight off invading substances). This result confirms an association between Earthing and the immune response, as was suggested in the DOMS study we mentioned a moment ago.

The Polish researchers concluded their report by saying that Earthing the human body influences human physiological processes and suggest that it may be a "primary factor regulating endocrine and nervous systems."

Again in 2011, the Sokals published the results of another study and hypothesized that Earthing's broad impact on the body's bioelectrical environment and electrolyte concentrations helps regulate "correct functioning of the nervous system" and "significantly influences" the electrical activity of the brain. In 2012, they further reported on a unique stability of the body's electrical functioning that occurs immediately and systemically upon grounding, as measured on various tissues of the body, including venous blood. Such changes disappear abruptly upon disconnecting the body from the Earth. The findings suggest that the nervous system and brain react instantly to grounding and operate more stably as a result.

THE EARTHING HYPOTHESES

The studies we have been describing have uncovered a simple but powerful fact: people who are grounded function better than they do ungrounded. They are, in fact, different. Based on the research, two scientists who have extensively studied and written about Earthing have made a number of intriguing hypotheses. They are James Oschman, Ph.D., and electrophysiologist Gaétan Chevalier, Ph.D.

The following is a summary of these ideas.

Living Longer and Better

Antiaging medicine involves the search for factors that can restore and maintain adequate energy resources and the circulation of vital energy throughout the body. This quest has been going on with humans throughout history. It's nothing new.

Our research clearly shows that grounding has a powerful influence on the delicate balance between health and illness, and looming behind that, the prospect of living longer and better. This antiaging prospect is clearly one of Earthing's most attractive aspects.

The dominant theory of aging—the concept of free-radical oxidative damage to the body—was first proposed by Denham Harman, M.D., of the University of Nebraska in 1956. The idea here is that aging results from the cumulative damage to the body produced by free radicals. These molecules can damage DNA, leading to mutations and disease. They are formed by metabolic processes in mitochondria, the "power plants" inside cells, and can gradually harm mitochondrial functioning and energy production throughout the body. They cause cross-linking of proteins, chemical reactions that interfere with normal enzyme activity. This is what causes skin to wrinkle for example. There is no way to prevent the formation of free radicals, because every breath we take and every morsel of food we eat feeds the natural mitochondrial production of energy and free radicals as a byproduct. Because of the constant threat of free radicals, we are encouraged to eat foods rich in antioxidants.

The living matrix, as one of its main biological functions, is set up to protect tissues from free-radical damage. It represents a natural, built-in antioxidant defense system. The matrix is all-pervasive, reaching into every corner of the body. If your matrix functions properly, and if you are connected to the Earth, any free radical formed anywhere in your body will be neutralized by mobile electrons from the Earth. This idea alone should motivate anyone to connect with the Earth as much as possible, day and night.

By understanding that the living matrix is a conductive fabric extending throughout the body, and that grounding connects this system to the Earth and an infinite source of free electrons, one can see that Earthing could prove to have far-reaching antiaging, antioxidant, and antiinflammaging effects. Long-term, controlled animal studies will enable us to verify or refute this profound hypothesis.

Research done in Germany has described the matrix in terms of a systemic reservoir of charges designed to maintain electrical balance and supply electrons in times of normal inflammatory need. Earthing provides recharging and keeps the reservoir full. Disconnection from the Earth dries up the reservoir.

A New Definition of "Normal" Immune Response

A common deficiency of electrons in the ungrounded body appears to distort and weaken the function of the immune system. But it can be readily restored to normal functioning by Earthing. The research suggests that Earthing may, in fact, create a whole new definition of what is a "normal" immune response.

As explained in Chapters 3 and 7, the inflammatory basis of disease has become a major focus of biomedical research. It is becoming widely accepted that chronic inflammation and chronic diseases, including so-called diseases of aging, are closely related. The classical inflammatory response may actually be an abnormal condition caused by separation from the Earth's readily available bank of free electrons. When the body is connected to the Earth, the classical signs and symptoms of inflammation are greatly reduced or absent, among them pain.

Promotes Healing of Injuries

The body forms an "inflammatory barricade" around sites of injury, where the immune system focuses on elimination of pathogens and damaged tissue. Free radicals involved in this process can spread from these sites and attack nearby healthy tissue, leading to chronic inflammation.

Earthing research gives the impression that free electrons can penetrate the barricade and thereby neutralize free radicals that have accumulated in pockets of inflammation. This ability appears to be a factor in accelerated healing.

A New Definition of "Normal" Physiology

When the body is connected to the Earth, a variety of beneficial physiological changes take place instantly. The studies that utilized a conductive patch placed on the bottoms of the feet and the palms of the hands made it possible to record the precise instant of connection to the Earth and document the sharp differences in various physiological parameters before and after grounding.

As scientific investigations continue, we expect to see countless more changes. The changes suggest that normal physiology may require a whole new set of ranges and definitions.

Restoring Your Internal Electrical Stability

The body utilizes Earth's electrical energy (ground) to maintain its internal electrical stability for the normal functioning of all self-regulating and self-healing systems. The modern way of life prevents contact with the Earth most of the time, creating electrical instability. This lack of stability results in body system dysfunctions that lead to inflammation, inflammaging, disease, and aggravation of existing disorders.

The Earth serves the human body as a source of energy similar to a power line feeding electrical energy into electrical equipment and appliances. It is widely accepted that equipment will not function well without a ground. The Earth also plays that role for living beings, including human beings. To read more technical information about the electrical effects produced by grounding, refer to Appendix A and B.

Resetting Your Biological "Clocks"

Biological clock systems are found, not only in humans and mammals, but in lower organisms as well, such as fish and insects. They are linked to survival. Although the human body packs several biological clocks (called peripheral clocks), researchers have found they are all under the control of a master clock located in the head, more precisely in the suprachiasmatic nucleus, a pair of distinct groups of cells in the hypothalamus.

One of the most important hypothalamic functions is to connect the nervous system to the endocrine system via the pituitary gland, the master gland of the body. Through hormonal secretions, it governs a multiplicity of activities affecting all body systems. Another function of the hypothalamus is to control the secretion of adrenocorticotropic hormone from the anterior pituitary gland, which in turn stimulates the secretion by the adrenal cortex of cortisol (the stress hormone). This system is so important for understanding the stress response that it is known as the hypothalamic–pituitary–adrenal axis.

The master biological clock receives its clues about prevailing light conditions from specialized cells in the retina. Signals about light conditions travel from the hypothalamus to the pineal gland, which controls the secretion of melatonin. Melatonin is secreted only in conditions of darkness.

The biological clocks control virtually all body system functions, including, of course, the wake-sleep circadian cycle.

From our research, we believe that not only light conditions but Earth's energy as well coordinates the various biological clocks regulating hormone flow in the body. The slow and gentle rhythms of the Earth's energy field are essential for maintaining these clocks. One example we have discussed is the day/night cortisol rhythm that is normalized when sleep is improved through grounding. Another example is the secretion of melatonin, which happens at night. Melatonin is widely known as a sleep-promoting factor. Since we have seen in our earlier studies that grounded people sleep better, we hypothesize that the rhythm of this hormone is also normalized when sleeping grounded. Any such normalization effect is important because melatonin is a powerful antioxidant, a major protector of the brain by preventing loss of brain cells by self-inflicted death. Given that a variety of neurodegenerative diseases, such as Alzheimer's disease, parkinsonism, and amyotrophic lateral sclerosis (Lou Gehrig's disease), have a free-radical component, it is assumed that melatonin may be useful in forestalling the consequences of these debilitating conditions and improving the psychological health of these patients. Researchers are postulating also that melatonin has several major functions that probably help to protect against psychiatric illnesses.

At any point on the surface of the planet, the Earth's energy potential fluctuates according to the position of the sun and the moon, creating cycles such as the circadian cycle. This understanding helps to explain how passengers, after long flights across many time zones, can reset their internal clocks to "local time," so to speak, and quickly reduce the effect of jet lag by going barefoot or grounding themselves after arriving at their destination.

Our overall working hypothesis is that grounding leads to a much greater physiological stability because the diverse bodily rhythms are coordinated not only with the light/dark cycle but with all the natural rhythms of the environment.

EARTHING AND YOUR GENES

Additionally, there is the likelihood that the influx of electrons in the body has an effect at the genetic level.

DNA, we are taught, represents the entire blueprint for the human body. Traditional genetics goes far in explaining how unique biological traits are inherited.

Until about ten years ago, it was thought that the way we live shouldn't directly affect the genetic traits passed to our children. However, so-called "epigenetic controls" have been discovered recently that influence whether and when a certain gene or set of genes are turned on and turned off when a person's environment changes. The term means "over and above the genes." Such influences do not alter the primary DNA sequence but operate at the level of the chromatin (the protein fabric of the nucleus) that surrounds the genes.

Researchers have identified a number of immediate early genes (IEGs) that respond within seconds to hours when something changes in one's environment. Evidence exists, in fact, that IEGs are so sensitive that words or thoughts can trigger adaptive changes in genomic expression. These genes regulate other genes, including those that operate the immune system. How you see and interpret the world around you selects which genes are going to be activated and modifies the readout to make proteins that best fit your environmental circumstances.

Remarkably, some of these epigenetic patterns can be passed from parents to children. The idea of epigenetic inheritance has led to a general reevaluation and intense study of how inheritance works.

For people searching for natural cures, Earthing is a dream come true. And now the emerging field of epigenetics implies a bonus effect: The remarkable self-healing mechanisms that seem to be activated by Earthing can affect not only ourselves but are likely to also be passed on to our children and their children. Earthing may well have an even greater impact than we have thought, by creating a beneficial ripple effect in the evolutionary process.

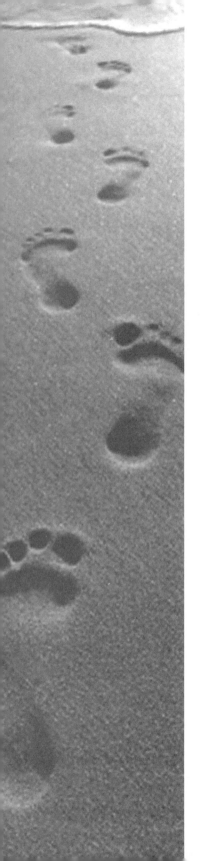

PART FOUR

The Earthing Chronicles

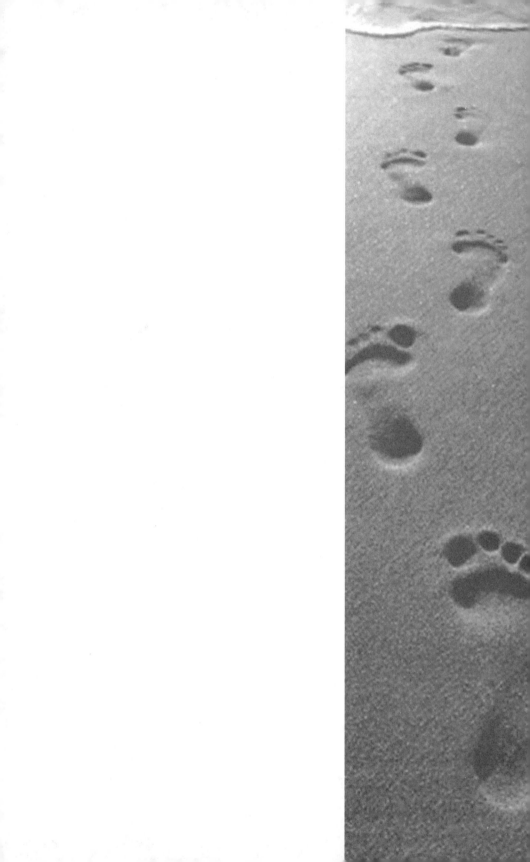

CHAPTER 9

Earthing 101:
How to Connect

We have told countless people to walk barefoot in their backyards, on the beach, in a grassy park, or on open ground where the surface is safe to walk on, and when the weather allows.

The feedback is inevitably one of surprise and delight.

Eileen McKusick, a sound therapist in Johnson, Vermont, expressed it this way: "I have been walking barefoot all summer, for the two-tenths of a mile back and forth to work, a few times a day, and pretty much anywhere else where I can go barefoot. I also walk around a big grassy field. I *love* being barefoot. I love, love, love it and I can't believe what a difference it has made in how I feel! More alive, more toned, more articulation in my feet, more settled emotions, greater overall well-being. Of all the things I have done for my health such as changing my diet, working out, taking supplements, getting bodywork, nothing has been as simple, inexpensive, easy, and enjoyable as taking off my shoes!"

Everybody knows that walking is a healthy way to get physical activity. During the day it's also a good way to get vitamin D. You get sunshine's vitamin D from above, *plus* the anti-inflammatory energy from the Earth below if you do it barefoot.

Physical activity. Vitamin D. Earth energy. It's a trifecta that gives new meaning to the term "power walking."

Of course, Earth's energy is there for your taking any time, day and night. It's free. Nobody has to pump it into your body like gasoline in a car. It's not a pill. It's not a potion. It's not an ointment. It's just something in the ground, on the ground, and from the ground right there beneath your feet. It's always been there and always will. You can have as much of it as you want. No limit.

Everybody talks about "green energy" these days. This is Earth energy —both the original and ultimate form of green energy for your body and well-being.

BAREFOOTING OPPORTUNITIES

Besides walking barefoot, you can, of course, ground yourself by sitting on the Earth or on a chair with your feet planted on the ground, while reading a book, listening to music, or just plain relaxing. For people with foot issues or tender feet, we recommend sitting in a comfortable chair with your bare feet placed directly on the Earth.

To make the Earthing experience most effective, dampen the soil or grass for added conductivity. Leave your feet squarely on the Earth and sit there for thirty or forty minutes. Actually, when any part of your body— your hands, forearms, legs, for example—makes contact with the ground, you are receiving the energy from below.

If you have the opportunity, connect with the Earth two or three times a day. The more time you put in, the more you benefit. The more compromised your health is, the more often and longer we recommend that you do this. But even in a half hour or so, you will have a remarkable shift. We have already measured some important physiological improvements within a half hour to forty minutes, and many more will come to light with continued research.

Many people have asked us about concrete. Is it conductive? The answer is maybe. Conductivity depends on the moisture level, and whether there is moisture through the concrete down to the ground. A dry concrete floor, or one with a moisture barrier beneath, or with a sealed or painted surface, will likely have little or no conductivity. Asphalt is made from petrochemicals and is not conductive. The same goes for a wood or vinyl surface.

Water-wise, wading or swimming in the ocean is a great recreational form of grounding. Saltwater, rich in minerals, is highly conductive, and actually several hundred times more so than freshwater. Conductivity depends on the concentration of minerals in the water. So lake water is much less conductive than saltwater. And pool water is likely less than that. A plastic kiddie pool would not be conductive because the plastic would insulate the water from ground contact.

The amazing thing about Earthing is that it is so simple and fundamental. James Oschman, the energy-medicine expert, reports on new technologies emerging every day and is often asked to examine them and explain how they work. "What is most profound about Earthing," he says, "is the element of simplicity. I once attended a meeting on the East Coast, and one of my colleagues came in from the West Coast. She had a bad case of jet lag. I told her to take her shoes and socks off and step outside

Tree Hugging—Are You Grounded?

We've also been asked many times if tree hugging is a form of Earthing. The answer again is maybe.

- Trees are made of wood, an insulating substance. If you touch the dry bark of a tree, you are likely not grounded. Unless the tree is wet or you touch the sap of the tree, which comes from the ground, hugging a tree will likely not result in a significant transfer of the Earth's electrons.

- The soil under a tree is generally more moist than exposed soil, so if you are barefoot, you would likely be quite grounded whether you were in contact with the tree or not.

- If you hold the leaf of a tree or plant firmly between your fingers, you are grounded. The sap is very close to the surface. But you won't have the same effect from a dry leaf.

- If you touch the green stem of a plant, you are grounded.

- Trees and plants are living, grounded organisms. They resonate with their own frequencies and energy, and they also have their own "umbrella effect" as we describe in Chapter 8 on pages 76–77. This may also account for a calming, positive experience standing under a tree, or touching and hugging it.

Our recommendation: Yes, go hug a tree, touch a stem, or hold a leaf. They are alive and full of energy. Just watch out for the ants!

on the grass for fifteen minutes. When she came back in, she was completely transformed. Her jet lag was gone. That is how fast grounding works. Anyone can try it. If you don't feel well, for whatever reason, just make barefoot contact with the Earth for a few minutes and see what happens. Of course, if you have a medical problem, you should see a doctor. But for ordinary aches and pains, digestive or respiratory problems, or sore muscles, there is nothing that comes close to grounding for quick relief. You can literally feel the pain begin to drain from your body the instant you touch the Earth."

For many people, it may not be practical or possible to connect barefoot or bare-skinned with the Earth. The weather may be lousy and the prospect of freezing one's tootsies is hardly appealing. Or if the weather is good, contemporary living is so fast-paced that a meaningful hookup with the Earth may not be possible. There may not be time for a "barefoot break" during the daily routine. Or the thought of going barefoot may just not be appealing.

You would be surprised to know, however, that there is something of a "barefoot movement" going on. A lot of people are thumbing their noses at convention and going unshod for significant portions of their daily life.

A 2009 article in the Toronto *Globe and Mail* said that shoelessness is catching on—big time. Jennifer Yang wrote that "the Facebook fan page 'Being Barefoot' boasts more than two million fans, and . . . is one of the fastest-growing pages on the social networking site, according to a trend-tracking website, Inside Facebook. Across the Internet the 'barefoot lifestyle' is booming, with adherents turning to websites such as the Society for Barefoot Living (www.barefooters.org), with more than 1,200 members."

As far as the winter is concerned, one barefooter whom Ms. Yang interviewed was a sixty-four-year-old retired autoworker from southern (that's an important climate distinction in Canada) Ontario who has been mostly shoeless for fifteen years. "He even pads around barefoot during the winter," she wrote, "though he draws the line at temperatures below minus 18." That's zero Fahrenheit, and at that point, "he reluctantly slips on flip-flops." He, like most of the other shoeless converts, says that shoelessness feels more natural and healthier.

Comfort and naturalness aside, what's interesting about the current barefoot boom is that before the Earthing book was published in 2010 most of these unshod enthusiasts were unaware that they were picking up healing energy from the Earth. Since the book, its translation into multiple languages around the world, along with the publication of many articles and blogs about Earthing, these same individuals and a growing number of new enthusiasts are going out barefoot precisely for health reasons. Many of them have told us in words of this nature: "It felt great to be barefoot when I was a kid, and it feels great to do it again as an adult, but now I know why."

In the past, we all sat, stood, walked, and slept with conductive contact to the Earth. It was part of ordinary, daily living. Now, nobody in our industrialized society except Scouts, soldiers, backpackers, and backyard pajama-partyers sleep on the ground anymore.

One way to address the personal energy deficit that clearly exists as a result of our physical separation from Earth is to develop methods capable of being used while sleeping and sitting for prolonged periods.

BAREFOOT SUBSTITUTES

During more than fifteen years of scientific research and experimentation, Clint Ober utilized a variety of indoor conductive systems, including bed mats, sheets, sheet-like sleeping bags, and EKG patches. These and other continually evolving designs served also to accommodate an increasing demand for "barefoot substitutes" by people hearing about the benefits of Earthing. Such products are connected by a wire to a ground rod placed directly in the Earth or plugged into the ground port of a grounded electrical outlet. They can be utilized during sleep, work, and relaxing indoors.

All such paraphernalia do nothing restorative by themselves. They are simply conductors of the Earth's natural energy to the body when you are indoors or unable to go barefoot outdoors. The Earth does the magic. They replicate standing barefoot or lying directly on the Earth. They do not "run" on electricity. We like to think of them as extension cords connecting you to the Earth. With any of them, your body is immediately brought to the same electrical potential as the Earth.

Grounded Sheets

Sleeping on a conductive half or full sheet has proven to be a highly popular and effective way of grounding the human body. Contact with the Earth during the third of our lives we spend sleeping yields great benefits. Sleep is the time when the body rests and recovers from the stresses of daily activities. If we do not sleep well, the recovery process works inadequately, making us susceptible to stress-related problems. As these problems worsen, they can further interfere with sleep, making the situation even worse. This cycle of discomfort, stress, and insomnia can be readily reversed and improved in many cases by sleeping grounded. Some people have told us they have thrown out their sleeping aids after they started sleeping grounded.

One woman described her experience thusly: "It's as if there is a big bulge in the wire carrying the Earth itself full of flowers, green grass, and animals, right into my bed. I feel as if I am lying there surrounded by Nature."

Some years ago, a variation of the grounded sheet called the "recovery bag" was created for Tour de France cyclists and other athletes in order to accelerate recovery from extreme physical activity. It provides a cocoon-like Earth contact effect, where users slip between the top and bottom sheet, as they would a sleeping bag. The bag has also become popular for travel and general in-home use.

Looking to the future, it is our expectation that the mattress and bedding industry will see the obvious appeal of embracing grounding technology. We expect the industry to step up with a wide array of products, including a grounded mattress described on the following page.

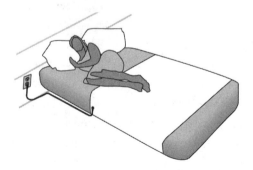

Figure 9-1. Sleeping on
conductive
half sheet.

Grounded Mattress

A grounded mattress is a natural sleep and health aid. People buy a new mattress every seven or eight years. So why not a conductive one? In addition to comfort and rest, you would experience improved health and less pain—as you sleep! Just lie down and go to sleep, and let Mother Earth do her magic!

Like conductive sheets and other barefoot substitutes, such a grounded mattress would be connected to a ground rod outside or through a properly grounded outlet in the bedroom. A simple conductive sheet, without a snap for a wire connection, could be used over the mattress so that it makes contact with the conductive fabric in the mattress. Since mattresses are home delivered from the stores where they are purchased, it would be simple for a delivery person not only to set up the mattress but also to check for proper grounding and connect it up.

The grounded bed should be the next big thing in the mattress industry. It should, in fact, be the new standard for mattresses.

Grounded Mats

Conductive mats are used in a variety of ways. Placed on a desktop, a mat can serve as a mouse pad, conducting through bare-skin contact with your forearms or wrists. Placed on the floor at your desk or in front of your favorite reading or TV chair, you simply put your bare feet on the mat. Thin socks will work as well.

The mats can also be placed on the bed, over your regular bottom sheet. You merely have to make bare-skin contact. Normal perspiration through thin layers of clothes, such as socks and pajamas, also permits varying degrees of conductivity.

Conductive mats have also been produced for yoga.

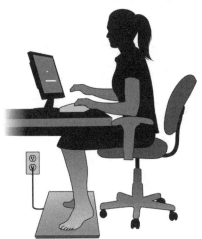

Figure 9-2. Floor mat.

A dense inlay of carbon particles or silver fibers gives the mat conductivity when connected.

Grounded Patches and Body Bands

Many of our scientific experiments have utilized electrode patches similar to the kind used by doctors for EKGs, EEGs, and other electrical activity diagnostics. The conductive patches can be attached near an injury or a wound, or an area of acute pain, to accelerate the healing process and reduce local inflammation and discomfort. Athletes have found them to be especially effective against common injuries and strains.

After experiencing quick pain relief, several participants in early grounding studies referred to the patches as "magic pain patches."

Some individuals, seeking concentrated relief for local pain (for example, in the arm, shoulder, or knee), have wrapped their grounded sheets around the affected area. This is somewhat similar to using a grounded electrode patch and sticking it on or near a wound or a site of pain.

We regard the grounded patches as a highly potent clinical aid that physicians may consider in the treatment of pain.

Another useful and flexible application is an adjustable conductive band placed around the wrist or ankle. It can be used in bed, while working at the desk, relaxing in a chair, and even while doing yoga.

Grounded Pet Pads

Conductive mats and pads for pets have been tested and found to provide improvement of pain, energy, stamina, flexibility, and stress. See Chapter 15 for more details.

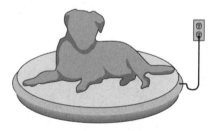

Figure 9-3. Dog on conductive pad.

Grounded Shoes

This is not a new principle. Grounded shoes are used in the electrostatic discharge industry to prevent buildup of static electricity in the body that could damage delicate electronic parts and chips.

Publication of the *Earthing* book inspired the development of a variety of flip-flops and sandals for everyday use by several American companies. Such grounded footwear is designed with conductive soles or inserts so that walkers can receive the Earth's energy without concern for stepping on barefoot hazards like glass and animal waste.

As Earthing becomes more popular, we expect shoe manufacturers to recognize a massive global-market opportunity for many grounded varieties of daily shoe wear: casual, sporty, work, recreational, and dress. In northern zones during the winter, conductive shoes and boots would give people an opportunity for outdoor Earthing under conditions when few people will venture forth barefooted.

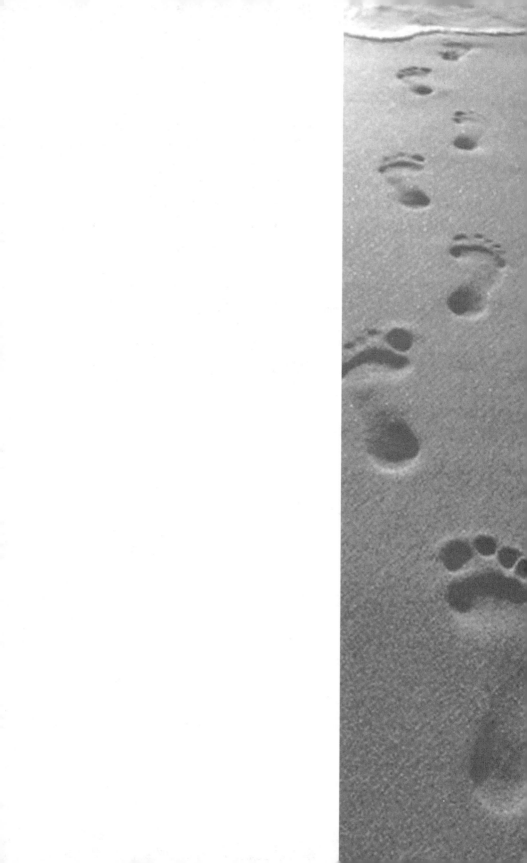

CHAPTER 10

Fifteen Years of Earthing: Clint Ober's Observations

Since 1998, I have been invited into the homes of probably several thousand people and reconnected them to the Earth. I have grounded newborns, kids, young adults, midlifers, seniors, and centenarians, and individuals deathly ill for whom the medical system had no more fixes to offer. Some understood what I was doing. Most didn't. They just understood later that they felt better and had less pain.

Earthing produces an amazing grassroots ripple. "Can you please do this for my mother or sister or father or friend?"

I've heard that many times from people who suffered for years with severe pain. Anyone who goes from pain to less pain or no pain, from fatigue to energy, from lack of mobility to more mobility, wants all their loved ones and friends to feel the same way.

"Oh, my God," they will say. "I didn't have to do anything. I didn't have to change my diet or exercise or take a pill. Just go to sleep."

I remember one case in which I grounded a mother at the request of her daughter, whom I had previously grounded. The older woman had suffered from chronic pain in the hips for more than ten years. I placed two grounded electrode patches on her feet. After about twenty minutes or so, she said she had to get up to go to the restroom. So I took the patches off. As she raised herself off the chair, she let out a scream. I got a real scare. I thought something had gone wrong.

"No," she said, "my pain is gone."

Dramatic as that sounds, I've heard it many times over the years. It is a common refrain of people being reconnected to the Earth after being disconnected perhaps for a whole lifetime.

The degree of gratification I have had seeing people lose their pain and feel better is beyond description. This is what has kept me going every day on an adventure that has been exhausting, challenging, and, at times, quite lonely. My joy has trumped the fatigue and time involved in trying to educate people about Earthing. Again and again.

After all these years, it is clear beyond any doubt that Earthing is safe and that many conditions and symptoms respond positively to the natural energy of the Earth. It is also clear to me that this connection with the Earth is *the* missing link for restoring red-bloodedness, hardiness, and health back into a society where the level of all of those has been plunging in recent years.

People often ask if Earthing will help them with certain health symptoms. Just as you can't direct healthy food, air, or water to create specific desired results in one function or part of your body, your body takes the natural energy from the Earth and uses it as needed. Often, people tell me of surprising "side benefits."

I strongly believe also that Earthing is not just to remedy health issues already present but also to assist our bodies in staying healthy. This is about the most natural form of prevention and antiaging medicine you can find.

Neither I, nor the researchers and doctors I have worked with, have a full understanding of the depth of physiological changes that occur with Earthing. We are scratching the surface of a great new paradigm that hopefully others, with greater resources, will be inspired to explore.

This I do know: Consistently reconnecting with the Earth restores a natural source of energy to your body that has been missing in your life. This missing energy may be the core cause of chronic inflammation and pain in your body, a malfunctioning nervous system, or some unresolved personal health issue. When you reconnect, and stay reconnected, all kinds of wonderful things can happen.

My observations over the years attest to a seemingly boundless potential for Earthing to help prevent and alleviate both common and uncommon health issues.

COMMON SYMPTOMS THAT IMPROVE

In general, people feel a greater sense of well-being when they are grounded. The sicker the individual, the more striking the gains. Older folks rapidly feel the spark of improved circulation and energy. Color, vitality, and outlook on life are transformed. Earthing helps circulation significantly. That's obvious to me after seeing countless gray faces brighten up with color from better blood flow. The first thing I've noticed—within minutes—with a lot of people is a change in their color. There's more color in their face or extremities. If the extremities are cold, they tend to warm up. "There's something going on down there," people have often told me after ten or fifteen minutes. Swollen joints and varicose veins subside. Some with many health issues are frequently different people after just a week or two of Earthing. Sure, they will still have those same issues, but they are getting better. One or more sources of pain are being reduced. They become more functional. Often they have told me, "I have my life back again."

Many women with menstrual issues have confided to me—a man and a stranger in their lives—that their periods are smoother after they started Earthing. I was once speaking at a health conference and was having a chat with a doctor and his wife afterward. I noticed that the wife had a painful look on her face. I asked her if she was okay. She said openly that it was PMS. I asked her if she would let me see if grounding could help her. I sat her down nearby, where I was demonstrating Earthing, and applied a grounded electrode patch for fifteen minutes on the palm of her hand. At the end of that time, she had a different look on her face. She said most of her discomfort had cleared up. The next day the doctor called me to say that his wife had felt so good that she was exercising on the mini-trampoline in their home. Usually, he said, she was down for a week.

Women in midlife often describe less discomfort from typical hormonal swings with grounding.

The main thing I have seen with children is a rapid calming effect. After grounding kids, parents are usually quite eager to have them traipsing around barefoot in the backyard. Nowadays, the first thing a kid will do in the morning is put on his or her shoes and the last thing at night is take them off. So they are ungrounded pretty much all the time, and this contributes, I believe, to a lot of the new health and emotional problems that kids have today, and it's another factor to add to the list of causes such as junk food and lack of exercise, and being exposed to long hours of television, computers, and video games.

Many experts say that kids—and adults as well—need to get out in Nature more and are healthier and better adjusted if they do so. Stress levels fall within minutes of seeing green spaces, one authority said. I second that, and I would add one more thing: Whether you go out into the countryside or your own backyard, go out barefooted wherever safe and possible. The stress level will drop even more.

People who sleep grounded are calmer, more energetic, and less stressed during the day. They wake up with less stiffness and soreness in the morning.

People with asthma and other respiratory ailments like bronchitis and emphysema breathe better. I've seen this often with children who have asthma.

Headaches often become less intense and frequent, and sometimes go away altogether.

If you have heartburn, go outdoors and plant your feet on the ground for twenty minutes and see what happens. Heartburn and acid reflux benefit from grounding.

Earthing has a stabilizing effect on the nervous system. One striking example of the healing potential on the nervous system was described to me by an acupuncturist who reported that after sleeping Earthed for a year, the mild and infrequent partial seizures she'd had for fifteen years seemed to have stopped.

If you have constipation, grounding may make you regular. It has done so for many people. Some individuals have told me they were able to discontinue laxatives.

I have seen many people with debilitating arthritis who have dramatically improved. I saw this right from the very start.

For individuals who are bedridden, a grounded bed sheet can reduce or eliminate bedsores. Hospitals need to ground their patients!

Eczema and psoriasis improve. So does dry skin. And dry, itchy eyes.

Food and pollen allergies improve and sometimes even clear up. Faulty immune systems seem to work better. By connecting with the Earth, it's as if you press a button on the immune system—like on a computer—

that switches disabled to enabled. I know this from firsthand experience. Years ago, when my kids were growing up, they would bring every virus and bug home from school, and I would inevitably catch what they got. In the years since I became grounded, I've had a few colds but that's about it. I used to suffer from pollen allergies, with a particular sensitivity to juniper. When the junipers blossomed, I would have difficulty breathing for weeks. Certain foods would cause red blotches on my throat. If I ate strawberries, I would break out with something like hives. Oranges gave me canker sores. There were long stretches of time when I was living off drugstore allergy remedies just to be somewhat comfortable. One doctor told me to stop eating wheat and grains with gluten. I don't have any of that anymore. I eat everything. I don't have any problem with juniper or pollens.

HOW FAST DOES EARTHING WORK?

There's no guarantee you will have an overnight healing like some of the people in the stories you will soon read about. It may take a while. You won't know until you do it—and stay with it. But I'll tell you this: I have seen plenty of people near death make comebacks that surprised their doctors, or who experienced a better quality of life before they passed away. And people who stay grounded just don't get sick—or as sick as they might normally do. They heal and their energy comes back faster.

People who ground themselves usually say they feel better within an hour, in many cases twenty minutes, whether they are walking or sitting barefooted, or are connected to the Earth through a conductive sheet, mat, or electrode patch. The research shows instant changes in physiology and significant improvements in the body's electrical activity inside a half hour or forty minutes.

I have seen some people with tension headaches have rapid relief, within five minutes. Others, such as someone with a chronic condition like arthritis, may take a half hour or so to notice some level of pain relief. But relief of pain and symptoms, in varying degrees and depending on what condition is involved, is a common response. The speed at which this occurs also varies from person to person. Relief can be significant, subtle, rapid, gradual, total, or partial.

I have found that lasting changes in stress, sleep, pain, and body rhythms occur when people stay connected to the Earth for longer periods of time on a continual basis. Nighttime sleep, when the body is most receptive to healing, appears to be an ideal time for Earthing. What better time for a natural healing when it occurs effortlessly while you sleep?

WHEN YOU STOP YOU LOSE THE BENEFITS

If you have chronic inflammation and you ground yourself for a period of time, and then stop, the body will usually sooner or later revert back to its previous ungrounded status. I have seen this regression happen with people and animals alike.

Many people report that the effects of Earthing continue with longer use. It is important not to give up too soon. You are plugging yourself into an energy source that is part of Nature's design. Your body's electrical system—that controls every cellular function—will function better when you reconnect.

EARTHING AND MEDICATION

Earthing improves the way the body functions in so many ways and it may, as a result, influence the requirement for medication. Many people have told me they have been able to reduce their dosage. I advised them, as I do anyone, that if you are involved in any medical treatment program it is best to inform your doctor about grounding. It is highly unlikely that he or she will have any knowledge of Earthing. This is all so relatively new.

If this is your situation you may want to show them this book. In any case, be alert to any symptoms that might reflect a medication overdose. Earthing doesn't interfere with medication. But your doctor may need to adjust the level you are taking. When undergoing routine medical testing, be alert to possible and surprising improvements in your results. Be sure your doctor addresses any changes that occur. Some results may indicate improved functioning and suggest lowering a dosage or even eliminating a medication.

For more information on Earthing and medication, see Appendix C.

EARTHING AND DETOXIFICATION

Some individuals with chronic inflammation, fibromyalgia, fatigue, anxiety, and depression, or who take multiple pharmaceutical drugs, may feel achiness, malaise, or flu-like symptoms initially grounding at night. They may, of course, actually have the flu, which has nothing to do with Earthing. But if not, such initial roughness may likely be due to a healing response promoting the release of toxins. As toxins pass through and out of the system, some temporary roughness may be experienced. When this happens, it is advisable to drink extra water to help flush out wastes. Another option is to cut back on the grounding and start with perhaps an hour a day, and then slowly increase your exposure. This approach gives your body a chance to adjust more slowly to the Earth's energy.

THE TINGLING SENSATION

People sometimes report feeling a tingling sensation in their body the first few times they are grounded at night. It is not unpleasant. And don't worry: You are not being electrocuted! You are simply feeling the Earth's natural, healing energy coming into your body. The tingling is related to the initial reenergizing, resynchronizing, and normalizing effects that this transfer of energy generates. The sensation usually diminishes and goes away after a few sessions of Earthing. It may be felt again once the individual resumes Earthing after stopping for some time. Sometimes the energy can create a feeling of achiness in parts of the body that are compromised, for instance, in the legs and feet of patients with diabetes who have poor circulation. As the extremities become energized, the experience initially may be felt as achiness or as fleeting cramps.

THE MALE CONNECTION

A number of men have described having better erections as a result of sleeping grounded. This might be a byproduct of improved circulation. Older men may also find themselves making fewer trips to urinate at night, due likely to reduction of prostate inflammation and deeper sleep.

EARTHING IS DOSE-RELATED

The longer you ground yourself in your daily life, the more stable, energetic, and robust your body functions and the greater your ability to heal. Some people describe symptoms disappearing or improving dramatically after just a few nights of sleeping grounded. Others say that symptoms and energy improve gradually, then reach a plateau and stay at that level as long as they continue grounding themselves. Some, after sleeping grounded through the night, will feel better and will have more energy or less pain when they awake but at midday may not feel as good.

As far as this last example is concerned, my experience indicates that the person simply needs to be grounded longer—the more time, the better—during the day.

This point was demonstrated dramatically in the case of one young woman who suffered with lupus, an autoimmune disease. She experienced substantial reduction of her symptoms when sleeping grounded for up to eight hours a night. She wanted to feel even better. So she used grounded floor and desk mats at her computer workstation and was able to often log up to eight hours more of Earthing. Her forearms were in contact with the desk mat as she worked, and she took off her shoes while at her desk. The additional hours made a big difference. In her case, Earthing during sleep was good, but sixteen hours of Earthing throughout the whole day was super-good.

The whole thing goes back to nature and the way our bodies were designed—in a grounded state, pretty much 24/7. If you sleep grounded, that's wonderful. That means, though, that your immune system is still in an ungrounded state for sixteen hours a day. If you can extend your hours of Earthing you stand to benefit even more, particularly if you have serious health issues.

Many individuals have told me about quantum leaps of improvement after extending their grounding hours into their active day. Earthing really has a dose-related effect. The longer you do it, the better.

Dale Teplitz, a health researcher who has worked with me on several of the studies and introduced Earthing to many people, uses a food analogy to help illustrate this point.

"People who eat junk food their entire life are depleted of many essential nutrients," she says. "Their health suffers as a result. If all of a sudden, they eat one healthy meal, they can't expect to have lasting benefits. But if they continue to eat healthy, over time the body gradually takes those elements and creates a healthier person. We humans have been disconnected from the Earth for our whole lives. We are depleted of the health-sustaining energy of the Earth. As with eating healthy, the longer we reconnect with the Earth, the more the body responds with improved health."

A single dose of walking on a sandy beach or sitting barefoot in your backyard will make you feel good for a while, but the effect won't last long. It's another thing if you can pursue such activities on a daily basis. Similarly, if you sleep grounded one night you will likely sleep better that night and feel more rested in the morning. But if you can routinely sleep grounded you are giving your body a major boost—a rock-solid foundation for maintaining health and a weapon for combating illness. And beyond that, some people will benefit still more from additional hours of grounding, particularly individuals with chronic inflammatory disorders.

Many people have asked over the years if it is harmful to get "too much" grounding. The question is understandable, but there is no evidence of getting too much. To me, it's like asking if a tree is getting too much of the Earth that it is rooted to. We are of the Earth and all our ancestors lived around-the-clock connected to the Earth. It's totally natural and, I think, unnatural and unhealthy not to be connected. Our bodies know exactly what to do with what the Earth provides for us. When we connect to the Earth, the amount of electrons we absorb and utilize is governed by the amount the body needs to balance its bioelectrical state.

Maximum benefits come when individuals live grounded around the clock or for a good chunk of a twenty-four-hour period. Our modern world, however, has become largely plasticized and insulated, keeping us separated from the Earth's healing energy. Hopefully, in the near future, we will re-evolve into a grounded society through access to conductive homes, offices, schools, bedding, furniture, and footwear.

Our contemporary fast-paced lifestyle, filled with chronic stress, poor eating choices, and lack of physical activity, has created a sick society.

Enjoyment of life is eroded. Personal and governmental resources are hemorrhaged. Earthing doesn't stop the bad habits, but it offers a natural remedy for halting some of the bleeding and the suffering. It is not a do-it-once-and-you-are-cured thing. Nor is it a cure-all. Rather it is a safe, effective, new-old paradigm that truly deserves thorough exploration and exploitation as a primary health and healing tool.

CHAPTER 11

The Cardiovascular Connection: Steve Sinatra's Perspective

During decades in cardiology practice I have witnessed remarkable advances that give doctors ever-greater ability to improve and save the lives of patients. However, I regard the most impressive breakthrough of all as something about as low-tech as you can get—the simple proposition of reconnecting to the Earth.

To be sure, Earthing research is in its bare infancy, but I've seen enough to know beyond doubt that our own planet offers us something massively protective, preventive, and therapeutic. Moreover, it is something easily "harnessed" by people everywhere. Nothing else I know can produce the same magnitude of systemic effects that includes reduced inflammation, improved blood electrodynamics, and a stabilization of the nervous system's influence on the heart. These are clearly major across-the-board benefits for common cardiovascular issues like high blood pressure, coronary artery disease, arrhythmias, and diabetes.

In addition to my own observations, I can also draw some assurance knowing that countless barefoot and much-closer-to-Nature generations before us were pretty much free of cardiovascular disease. Today, it ranks as the No. 1 disease killer in the Western world and is rising fast in the developing world where it was previously uncommon.

What follows is a roundup of information that has me so excited about Earthing's cardiovascular impact and potential.

THE EARTH AS A NATURAL BLOOD THINNER

Blood is a complex fluid. It carries a critical cargo of oxygen, nutrients, metabolic wastes, and clotting factors. You don't have to be a doctor to understand the importance of good flowing blood that's able to pass through thousands of miles of tiny blood vessels to service all the nooks and crannies of your body.

Viscosity is a term that refers to the water and solid content of plasma and how well, or not so well, the blood flows through this system. Thick, sludgy blood doesn't move through efficiently to deliver the goods and carry out the wastes. Cells and tissues underperform that are thus underserved. They become more vulnerable to toxicity and inflammation. I have always told my patients I want to see blood like the consistency of flowing wine, not sludgy like ketchup.

Thick blood is inflamed blood, predisposing you to red blood cell aggregation and abnormal clotting. This is the sort of blood that I became increasingly aware of in my patients after many years of medical practice: sludgy, sticky, hypercoagulable blood unable to slip effectively through the circulatory system, and causing the heart to work harder. Medical research is full of studies linking such blood to common cardiovascular ills.

Enter Earthing.

In 2008, I invited colleagues to my home in Connecticut to participate in an unusual experiment. There were twelve of us. We were clinical physicians, Ph.D.s working in the medical field, nurses, artists, a personal trainer, an attorney, and Clint Ober.

The experiment involved taking a drop of blood before and after forty minutes of grounding via EKG patches connected to the Earth, and then examining the unstained blood under a darkfield microscope. These microscopes, used by many doctors, particularly in the field of alternative medicine, divert light through the optical system so that details appear light against a dark background. The technique allows viewing of "live time" cellular dynamics and conditions of blood not normally analyzed through routine tests.

The pictures shocked us. All the before-grounding samples, except one, revealed various degrees of red "ketchupy" blood. See Figure 11-1 on the opposite page. The sole exception, the sample with the best blood of anyone present, was Clint Ober's—someone who has been consistently Earthing himself day and night for years!

The after-grounding pictures showed dramatic changes. There were considerably fewer formations of red blood cells associated with clumping and clotting. The blood appeared more thinned out. From a cardiology standpoint, if you can thin typical ketchup-like blood of heart patients and people with diabetes in the direction of the consistency of wine, as our simple experiment suggested, you remove a colossal risk factor.

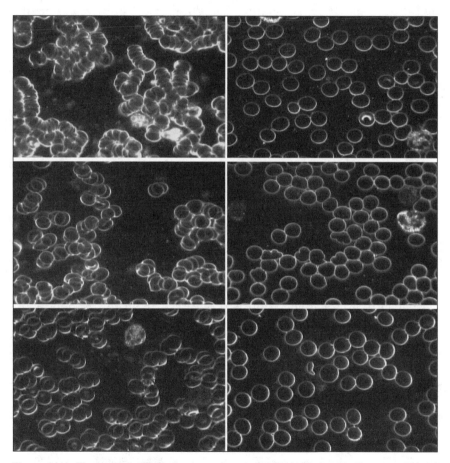

Figure 11-1. The reproductions above represent darkfield microscope images of blood taken from three individuals in attendance at Dr. Sinatra's house just before and after forty minutes of grounding. The before images are on the left, the after on the right. The pictures clearly show a dramatic thinning and decoupling of blood cells.

MORE EVIDENCE—THE ZETA POTENTIAL CONNECTION

The experiment inspired a formal study to investigate further whether Earthing can indeed influence red blood cell clumping. Electrophysiologist Gaétan Chevalier, Ph.D., biophysicist James Oschman, Ph.D., cardiologist Richard Delany, M.D., and I designed a study to measure not only blood clumping but also zeta potential, a term that describes the degree of negative charge on the surface of a red blood cell. Our blood cells operate electrically and this particular built-in feature enables the cells to repel each other and prevent unwanted aggregation. The stronger the negative charge, the greater the ability of the cells to repel each other and the better the flow. Zeta potential is not a familiar cardiology term, even though research linking it to cardiovascular function goes back to the 1950s.

For our study, we selected ten healthy individuals. They came individually to a health clinic and sat comfortably in a reclining chair while they were grounded for two hours. Electrode patches connected by wires to the Earth were placed on their feet and hands, just as had been done in previous studies. Blood samples were taken before and after two hours of continual grounding.

The analysis was surprising. We had expected a small improvement in zeta potential, perhaps 30 percent. Instead, we found an improvement of 270 percent on average! The results, published in 2013 in the *Journal of Alternative and Complementary Medicine*, indicated the discovery of a natural blood thinning effect, an option that should be of great interest for cardiologists as well as any physician concerned about the relationship of blood viscosity and inflammation.

The healthy range for zeta potential is between minus 9.3 millivolts (mV) and minus 15 mV, with an average of minus 12.5 mV. In our experiment, two hours of grounding improved the average zeta potential of the ten participants from a rather depressed level of minus 5.28 mV before Earthing to a healthy minus 14.26 mV afterward.

Blood closer to a zero zeta potential is more apt to be sludgy and thick, flow less freely, and have a greater risk of clumping and clotting. You'll see additional research on that in a moment, when I discuss diabetes.

Blood vessels are like highways. You want the traffic moving smoothly and fluidly. You don't want traffic jams. In our study, we exposed the blood samples to an electric field and observed, with the darkfield micro-scope, how much the red blood cells moved in a certain period of time before and after grounding. The red blood cells barely moved in the samples taken before. After grounding, they moved briskly along. In addition, we documented considerably fewer clumps of red cells in the after samples compared to the pregrounding samples. This response helped us understand why we frequently see people's skin turning pink soon after they become grounded. It's almost as if the floodgates of a dam are opened.

If Earthing affects blood electrodynamics like this, we believe it also affects cells throughout the body, and further supports our belief that grounded people have a different physiology than people who are ungrounded.

Relief from Peripheral Artery Disease Pain

Peripheral artery disease is a condition involving reduced blood flow to the extrem-ities. It occurs in 5 percent of adults older than fifty and in 20 percent above sev-enty. Among the common symptoms is pain in the legs.

H. M. Kearney, Ph.D., Webster, New York, retired historian: "I began sleeping grounded in 2010, virtually at the same time I was diagnosed with peripheral artery disease. My most immediate experiences were deeper sleep, fewer times getting up at night, marked improvement in overall energy, and much less discomfort on the treadmill.

"After several months, I was able for the first time in years to drive the 720-mile round trip to visit family without acute pain in my left leg, the more con-stricted extremity, and without discomfort in my right leg. Prior to Earthing, I had never completed the six-plus-hour journey each way pain-free. I was amazed!

"Equally amazing, as I enter my fourth year of Earthing, is that these pos-itive results have continued. Recent assessment of my condition indicated a slight decline but much less than my physician or I would have expected. Am I delighted? Absolutely! Traveling? Never leave home without my Earthing sheet."

THE NERVOUS SYSTEM–HEART CONNECTION

Perhaps one of the most overlooked Earthing dividends—and so beneficial in these stressful times—is the rapid calming influence that takes place within the autonomic nervous system (ANS) that regulates functions like heart and respiration rates, digestion, perspiration, urination, and even sexual arousal.

This effect may be one of the first, and possibly the first, of the major body systems that react to Earthing. It begins pretty much instantly. The ANS shifts from a typically overactive sympathetic mode, associated with stress, into a parasympathetic, calming mode. The sympathetic and parasympathetic systems are the two branches of the ANS.

Stress throws off the balance between the two branches. Too much sympathetic "arousal"—from stress—leads to the well-known "fight-or flight" mode, an alert and readiness state that humans automatically switch on when in imminent danger, like fighting in a battle. In today's world, unpredictable social, financial, and political events conspire to keep stress levels at an unhealthy high level as well. Many people live day-to-day in a state of physiological arousal. Whenever you can turn down the stress volume in your body, it's good for the heart and all the rest of you.

Revved-up sympathetic activity overwhelms the calming parasympathetic influence. The result, among other things, is a heightened risk of hypertension, arrhythmias, and even sudden death. One major yardstick of sympathetic overdrive is disturbance to heart rate variability (HRV), a measurement of nervous system balance on heart function.

HRV refers to imperceptible beat-to-beat alterations in heart rate. People with low variability are less able to "go with the flow" when faced with stress and are more prone to stress-related disorders, including cardiovascular disease. HRV is different than when your heart beats faster as a result of exerting yourself or becoming stressed, and slowing down when you relax. Variations of HRV are seen on electrocardiograms and sophisticated computer analyses. You can't feel the difference, but when you breathe in, your heart rate increases just ever so slightly. When you breathe out, it decreases ever so slightly.

HRV superbly indicates your ability to cope with both internal and external changes. It is, in fact, "the most accurate predictor of sudden death and the most accurate reflector of stress," according to Paul Rosch, M.D., president of the American Institute of Stress in New York City. "If you can alter HRV, that is, increase it, you can reduce the likelihood of stress-related disorders, including cardiovascular disease."

Exercise, tai chi, yoga, and meditation are examples of activities that improve ANS and HRV. You become more relaxed and you sleep better. This effect is precisely what many people report after they start Earthing and prompted another study that I conducted with electrophysiologist Gaétan Chevalier.

Earlier Earthing investigations (see Chapter 8) had demonstrated a marked alteration in a variety of biological parameters after about twenty to thirty minutes. Others in several days. Some showed even a dramatic change immediately at grounding (in less than a second or two). In the HRV experiment, we monitored twenty-eight men and women (average age, forty-eight) before, during, and after forty-minute grounding sessions while seated comfortably in a recliner chair. They were also monitored, for comparison sake, for an identical forty-minute period while sham grounded.

When grounded, there was an instant change in HRV that kept improving all the way to the end of the session, suggesting a greater benefit with time. There was no change in HRV when the same participants were sham grounded. The experiment, showing a positive trend in HRV, was published in 2011 in *Integrative Medicine: A Clinician's Journal.*

For individuals who experience anxiety, emotional stress, panic, fear, and/or symptoms of involuntary muscle contractions and spasms, including headaches, cardiac palpitations, and dizziness, Earthing appears to represent a promising strategy that can be felt rapidly.

Grounding research by Polish cardiologist Karol Sokal and neurosurgeon Pawel Sokal suggests that the Earth's energy likely plays a basic role in enabling the nervous system to adapt to the demands of the organism and the environment. As a cardiologist, I have repeatedly treated the human wreckage that stress—acute or chronic sympathetic overdrive—can exact. I have applied the best tools that both conventional and alternative medicine offers. Reconnecting the body to the Earth provides perhaps the most natural tool available anywhere.

Our study provided additional evidence demonstrating Earthing's potential to balance the nervous system, reduce the stress response, and support cardiovascular health. Such effects go beyond basic relaxation and may explain in part the repeated feedback from people experiencing lower blood pressure and improved arrhythmias after they start Earthing.

If there is a trend toward improved HRV in forty minutes, what will sleeping grounded routinely for six or eight hours do?

Here are several outstanding examples reported to me:

- After ten weeks, a seventy-three-year-old woman reported that her blood pressure went down by 10 points and she slept much better.

- A husband's snoring stopped and he slept better. The wife's blood pressure went down from 150/90 to 120/80 mm Hg after one night!

- One woman experiencing distressing skipped or extra heartbeats said that sleeping grounded eliminated them. Not only that, her husband's atrial fibrillation episodes stopped. He had been taking Coumadin, a popular blood thinner, for his condition and, in conjunction with his doctor, was able to reduce dosage.

Our study suggests that Earthing should be considered as a significant natural, cost-effective, and noninvasive intervention that positively impacts the ANS.

NEW HOPE FOR DIABETES

Diabetes is a global scourge of pain, suffering, and premature death that kills an estimated 3.4 million people a year—a number sharply on the rise. It contributes to arterial and nerve damage, heart attack, stroke, poor circulation, foot ulcers, lower limb pain and numbness, weakness in hands and feet, kidney disease, and vision problems.

A healthy diet, regular physical activity, and maintaining a normal body weight are widely promoted to prevent or delay type 2 diabetes, the most common form of the disease (90 percent of cases). We strongly believe that the increasing human disconnect from the Earth's natural surface charge is a major missing link here.

Since the mid-1900s there has been a proliferation in increasingly unnatural lifestyle practices, including sedentary work, less active time spent outdoors, and overeating nutrient-poor processed food full of refined carbohydrates. (See Plate 6 "Correlation or Coincidence?" on page 86.) These are driving forces for diabetes. But so, too, is the overlooked disconnect with Mother Earth.

Reconnection helps in a number of significant ways.

Reduction of Inflammation

One main component of diabetes involves a scenario where excess fatty tissue in the abdomen produces inflammatory chemicals that suppress insulin, a hormone that regulates the movement of sugar (glucose) in the cells. The body then becomes more resistant to insulin. This in turn produces more inflammatory chemicals and interference. Blood sugar rises. Add stress to the mix, and you further increase the level of inflammatory chemicals.

The influx of electrons from Earthing reduces chronic inflammation.

Electrical Stability in the Body

Earthing restores the body's electrical stability and has a major effect in restoring order to the normal functioning of all body systems.

Calming the Nervous System

Earthing calms the ANS and improves HRV. Abnormalities in HRV are regarded as early evidence of cardiovascular autonomic neuropathy, a widely overlooked complication of diabetes that damages nerve fibers supplying the heart and blood vessels. Such abnormalities disturb heart rate control and vascular dynamics.

Aiding Glucose Control

Among other things, poorly regulated glucose causes diminished elasticity of red cells and an increased tendency to aggregate. The result: thicker blood, poorer blood flow.

A growing awareness exists about the blood viscosity–cardiovascular disease connection, but the link between elevated viscosity and diabetes is largely overlooked even though it has been reported in more than fifty peer-reviewed scientific publications. Blood viscosity can be improved by eating less sugar, stepping up one's physical activity, and treating gum disease, a factor that promotes systemic inflammation, as measured by increased C-reactive protein (an inflammation marker) and fibrinogen, a sticky, fibrous coagulant in the blood that raises the risk of stroke.

Earthing helps control blood glucose. We have seen that effect in an unpublished yearlong laboratory study showing a small but significant reduction in the glucose level of grounded rodents compared to non-grounded animals. Two other biochemical markers, triglycerides and alkaline phosphatase, were also lowered, suggesting less risk of diseases linked to the metabolic syndrome, such as hypertension and diabetes.

Zeta Potential and Better Blood Flow

A fascinating 2008 study from the University of Calcutta in the medical journal *Biochimica et Biophysica Acta* reported for the first time on the zeta potential of red blood cells in diabetics. It's not a good picture. The researchers described "a remarkable alteration," specifically a progressive deterioration of zeta potential, most pronounced among diabetics with cardiovascular disease. The research revealed a parallel between poorer zeta potential and hypercoagulability.

"Blood becomes sludge so that it becomes increasingly difficult for the heart to pump, and the system becomes less efficient to perform the usual functions," they said, and recommended that zeta potential should be used as a measurement of cardiovascular disease in individuals with diabetes.

A few years earlier, this same group of researchers reported that high blood sugar causes oxidative damage to red blood cells and hemoglobin. Hemoglobin is the molecule in blood cells that carries oxygen from the lungs to the body's tissues and then carries out carbon dioxide. In 2008, the Indian researchers said that the high blood sugar also significantly alters the electrodynamics of the cells' outer membrane, thus increasing the potential for clumping.

Our zeta-potential study offers one intriguing explanation of how individuals with diabetes may benefit from Earthing. Clearly, though, everyone stands to benefit, not just diabetics. Zeta-potential improvement is one of the biggest effects of Earthing, and perhaps the biggest of all.

Prime Example: My Bookkeeper's Mother

In early 2010, the then eighty-one-year-old diabetic mother of my book-keeper, Jodie Mitchell, was having a terrible time. The woman, a retired school-bus driver, suffered with painful, throbbing legs that disturbed her sleep multiple times every night. She would arise exhausted and have to nap during the day. She frequently developed horrible sores on her legs that would take considerable time to heal, a common problem among diabetic patients, and the likely result of poor circulation.

She had developed a quarter-sized sore on her calf that did not respond to topical medicines. I suggested Earthing. Three weeks into sleeping grounded, the throbbing pain was almost gone. Jodie told me her mother was sleeping through the night, perhaps getting up once to relieve herself but no longer from pain. Her energy level had soared and the open sore was no longer open. It was covered with a new growth of pink skin and was healing.

In 2013, Jodie's mother's energy is still great! She has experienced no sores since. She stays grounded and has minimal leg pain.

In Plate 5 on page 85, you can see graphic pictures of how Earthing improves the circulation and leg sore challenge faced by people like Jodie's mother and other diabetics.

The Polish Experience

In Poland, cardiologist Karol Sokal and his neurosurgeon son Pawel have been documenting the various effects of grounding on the physiology for more than two decades. In a conversation with them, they shared the following details:

"We have seen good things with diabetes. We were able to withdraw insulin for some people because they achieved a reduction in their blood sugar just from walking barefoot. We found that in some cases the combination of medication and grounding could even push the glucose level too low.

"Imagine telling someone that if you go barefoot you may be able to reduce or withdraw your insulin . . . or some other medication! Yet this is what we found. It all depends on the level of glucose as to whether and when you can cut out the medication or reduce it. With oral medication, we observed that some people with diabetes could walk barefoot and not need antidiabetic drugs like Metformin.

"Here in Poland, you can't go barefoot outside throughout the year. You have to wait until late spring and summer. If people have stone or concrete floors in their homes, they can try to walk or sit barefooted on the floor. Doing that for a few hours a day, people are often able to reduce their medication within a few weeks. But not everybody can spend that kind of time barefoot, of course.

"One of our experiments with blood sugar showed that continuous grounding for three days and two nights was enough to decrease the level of glucose in patients with diabetes. The result was on the basis of twelve volunteers, six of whom were grounded. Further research with more people would be needed to see at what point sustained grounding could achieve a decrease in glucose enough to recommend that a doctor reduce the medication dosage. Perhaps a minimum of three nights may be enough for some people."

The Australian Experience

From David Richards, M.B.B.S., an integrative family physician in Iluka, New South Wales, we received the following detailed report on his experience with diabetes: "In my more than thirty years as a general practitioner, I've never had anything to offer patients for diabetic neuropathy. No doctor really has anything. All we can do is try to optimize blood sugar and control it. But that doesn't fix the problem of numb feet. Earthing has changed this dilemma altogether.

"In most cases, I have seen at least some improvement of foot numbness after an initial hour grounding session in my office where patients simply put their bare feet on an Earthing mat. Some have not been able to come back immediately but generally improvement lasts for as long as ten days after one session. The more they do, the better, though.

"One diabetic woman said that her numb feet had improved by 75 percent after that one session. She had never told me she had numb feet. After two sessions, her numbness was totally resolved. To date, the numb feet of twenty-one out of twenty-one patients are mostly resolved!

"I now deliberately target diabetics, even those without complications. I believe Earthing offers preventive benefit by counteracting inflammation and helping improve blood flow to all smaller vessels.

"In my practice, I personally draw blood and I have repeatedly observed the change in blood viscosity. One patient, whose neuropathy resolved, used to have blood that would clot in a normal-sized venesection needle before even making it to the blood tube. Since starting Earthing that doesn't happen anymore!

"The renal function of three kidney patients has returned to normal. One had been told by a kidney specialist that she would be on dialysis in three years. I started her on an Earthing program at home and when she next visited the specialist two months later she was told that perhaps she would need dialysis in five years. When I heard from her again, she said there 'was not much to report.' Her kidney function remains the same and if it remains stable she will probably *never* need dialysis. The other two patients are also stable and if they continue Earthing they will likely not need dialysis either.

"One of these patients likes to go fishing barefoot. He remarked how he had forgotten how sharp the rocks were and how hot the sand was! He can feel them now. He couldn't before.

"The other patient now describes the condition as 'slowly' progressive renal disease. I have never heard the term 'slowly' attributed to renal disease.

"The brother-in-law of a good patient of mine reluctantly tried Earthing. He is on dialysis. His specialist told him, 'I don't know what you are doing but keep doing it.'

"One patient with vascular disease now sleeps grounded. He chided me during an office visit: 'Why didn't you tell me about this years ago?' His usually cold feet are re-warmed within minutes of contact with the Earthing sheet.

"I have seen diabetic eye disease stabilize in two patients. Another, with glaucoma, reported visual improvement, 'like cling film being lifted from in front of the television screen.'

"Another individual with a leaking heart valve has experienced resolution based on a recent echocardiogram. His specialist can't explain it.

"Prior to Earthing, one diabetic patient experienced considerable depression. The depression has improved with twice-a-week Earthing in my clinic over several months.

"I find that medication needs generally are reduced after Earthing. One patient now only takes insulin if she is lax with her diet. Another has reduced daily insulin from 80 units down to 10 or 20 units. I actually warn patients to be alert for improvement and be prepared to reduce doses of some medications, such as blood pressure, thyroid, and glucose meds, and, in particular, blood thinners. For those on blood thinners, such as Coumadin, I do standard blood-clotting checks fortnightly [every two weeks] for about two months, and if the blood is stable, then do it monthly. I haven't encountered any issues.

"Earthing brings into the treatment equation an entirely unusual prospect. The majority of doctors expect deterioration in patients and the need to add more medication and/or to increase doses. Now, along with noticeable improvements and lowering medication, it seems to me that diabetics over a long period of time will also have less heart disease, less stroke, and better health as a result of Earthing.

"And not just diabetics. I started Earthing a new patient recently. She had spinal surgery twenty-seven years before and hasn't been able to flex her toes or feel her left foot/lower leg since the operation. She can now! If it weren't for Earthing, she might have spent the rest of her life carrying what she had always referred to as her 'dead leg.'

"I have male patients who after sleeping grounded tell me they can pee with more force. Presumably their age-related prostate swelling is somewhat better. Most feel calmer, sleep deeper, and generally feel better overall. I also see better wound healing and a concept quite unusual in my career: blood pressure and thyroid conditions improving.

"Medicine doesn't have many 'wow' moments. It is mainly logical thinking with little scope for being somewhat creative. Medicine plus Earthing has provided me lately with some spectacular wow moments."

THE BLOOD PRESSURE CONNECTION

Doctors don't know the precise cause of high blood pressure (also known as hypertension), but they know it affects a huge segment of humanity and is increasing at an alarming rate. A 2013 World Health Organization report says that complications of hypertension, such as heart attack and stroke, account for 9.4 million deaths worldwide every year and that in another decade, an estimated 1.56 billion people will be affected.

Over the years I have used a nondrug approach for prevention and therapy involving diet, supplements, mind/body techniques, and exercise. I found that mild high blood pressure is one of the easiest medical conditions to control without drugs or medical treatment. Individuals with severe high blood pressure and symptomatic kidney disease, a result of high blood pressure, need to take medication.

Earthing provides another major tool. I have frequently heard comments about improved blood pressure from people after they start Earthing. Some individuals have said that their doctors have been able to reduce their medication dosage, and, in some cases, eliminate medication altogether.

Here's a couple of examples:

- "My blood pressure, although still at the same dose of medication as before, runs at a consistently lower reading, something I haven't seen since I started medication ten years ago."

- "I have seen great results with my eighty-six-year-old mother . . . who has been on four medications for high blood pressures for many years. Her blood pressure went down to a point where we had to take her off her medication and she is now taking one new medication, which is not as strong."

Such comments have become routine, and easily understandable when you consider these Earthing influences:

- Improved circulation and electrodynamics of blood.
- A calming effect on the nervous system.
- A normalizing effect on cortisol, the stress hormone.
- Better sleep.
- Less inflammation and pain.

Earthing may, in fact, represent the easiest possible way to lower your blood pressure. You can do it in your sleep without a pill or anything else. The most dramatic drops we have observed have been associated with a reduction of pain and the anxiety and fear of chronic illness.

If you are hypertensive and taking medication, and you want to start Earthing, please consult with your physician. He or she may need to adjust and lower your medication accordingly. You may want to track your own blood pressure with a monitoring device at home and bring to your doctor a written record of your readings before and after grounding sessions.

Occasionally, people have reported increased blood pressure after they start Earthing. However, there is nothing about Earthing that can cause an increase. Blood pressure either comes down or stays the same. A rise in blood pressure is unrelated to Earthing and is likely related to overwhelming emotional stress or to someone stopping medication.

Clint Ober recalls the case of one male participant in an early Earthing study whose blood pressure was very high and stayed high during the eight-week duration of the study. "His numbers changed very little," Clint remembers. "He stayed around 160. Meanwhile, the blood pressure of all the other people in the study dropped. I asked the doctor involved in the study what was going on with that individual. He told me that the man was having serious financial problems."

Clint also cites the case of a man who had been Earthing for many years and who normally had a blood pressure in the 110 to 130 range. When his mate died, he jumped to 160 mm Hg and stayed there for almost eight months. When his son died suddenly of a heart attack, his pressure went up again and stayed up for quite a while despite many hours day and night being grounded. It was the severe trauma of the losses.

"In my experience, I have seen many people, and especially women, have significant reductions in their blood pressure. That happens because of Earthing's systemic effects. People have less pain and become happier."

ARRHYTHMIAS AND EARTHING

"Something is wrong with my heartbeat. Is it serious?"

Every cardiologist and family practitioner hears this question from frightened patients. It usually refers to arrhythmias, a common occurrence involving an irregular heart rhythm. In essence, your heartbeat goes off cadence. Arrhythmias can range from simple skipped heartbeats called premature ventricular contractions, or PVCs, to the more serious varieties like atrial fibrillation and malignant ventricular irregularities. They are frequently set off by emotional stress and turmoil that generate heightened sympathetic activity.

PVCs are generally benign arrhythmias involving skipped or extra heartbeats, or combinations of the two, that can also be generated by too much caffeine and alcohol, deficiencies of magnesium and potassium, and different cardiac conditions.

PVCs may occur when you settle down in bed, may wake you up in the middle of the night, or may grab your attention when walking the dog or working on the computer. They can happen randomly. If they happen frequently enough, they scare the heck out of you, and send you running to your doctor or even the emergency room.

PVCs involve a misfiring of the bundle of cells that regulate the electrical conduction to the ventricles, the two lower chambers of the heart due to some "irritability" of the heart muscle.

Earthing can be very helpful to curb PVCs, as the following story illustrates.

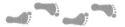

Wendy Saunders, Cincinnati, Ohio, mental health counselor: "I heard about Earthing several years ago and thought it might help improve my sleep. It didn't even occur to me that it might help my PVCs. Out of curiosity, I started Earthing with a wristband.

"At the time, I had been experiencing so many PVCs at night that they were interfering with my sleep. A Holter monitor recorded over 6,000 PVCs in a twenty-four hour period. Worst of all, I could feel nearly all of them.

"By the third night of sleeping grounded, I was astonished that I could not detect any PVCs. In addition, resting on my left side would usually trigger PVCs, but while sleeping grounded, I could rest on my left side without a problem.

"It's been about two and a half years now, and, although I have not been remonitored in this time, I haven't felt any PVCs at all. They are still gone. I sleep much better. My experience has been life-changing."

Atrial Fibrillation

Imagine living with a heart that vibrates, quivers, and races rapidly and erratically instead of beating in a steady, comfortable, and predictable rhythm. Atrial fibrillation is the medical name for this condition, the most common arrhythmia of the heart. Every year, 2 million or so people are diagnosed with "atrial fib" or "a-fib," as it is called for short. Although not by itself life threatening, it can lead to heart failure or stroke. For sure, it is scary. People frequently think they are having a heart attack.

In a normal heart rhythm, the upper chambers of the heart—the atria—contract in unison in response to an electrical signal generated by pockets of specialized cardiac cells called the sinus node. In patients with a-fib, however, the conduction becomes deranged and electrical signals scatter throughout the atria. Instead of contracting, the atria beat quickly and irregularly. This results in the loss of normal, synchronous pulsation and raises the risk of blood pooling and forming clots inside the chambers. Coumadin is usually prescribed to prevent clot formation.

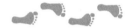

Bob Malone, Boulder, Colorado, financial adviser: "In 1996, after experiencing chest pain, rapid heartbeat, and flutter, I was diagnosed with a-fib. It's very scary. You don't know when the next episode is coming and whether you will survive. In my case, it was brought on by business stress. My work involves advice and decisions that affect people's lives.

"Medication kept the symptoms under control most of the time. When the meds were unable to control the wildness in my heart, I would have to get electroshock and jolt the heart back into a normal rhythm. I needed treatment like that every nine months or so. The meds were horrible. They took my energy down to zero. I've always been an active, creative guy, and I love the outdoors, and now this stopped me in my tracks.

"I started sleeping grounded in 2000. I went from not getting sleep and waking up frequently at night to getting good, solid sleep pretty much all the time. I later added a grounded floor mat while I was reading or watching TV, and even used one at the office where the stress level is pretty high.

"The incidents slowly started to stretch out. They went from days to weeks to months apart. I was slowly able to wean myself off medication. I had a flare-up in 2006, which I believe was related to the stress over the death of my brother. I had to take medication, but I haven't taken any since.

"In 2007, I went to the mountains for some fresh air and took an hour-and-a-half hike. My pulse was ranging between 115 to 130 beats per minute. In the process I got chest pain (angina), which happens whenever I exercise aggressively. Then it normally goes away at night when I sleep

Caution: Earthing and Blood-Thinning Medication

If you take Coumadin (warfarin) or other pharmaceutical anticoagulants, talk first to your doctor before grounding. Earthing has a blood-thinning effect, as described earlier. The combination of medication and Earthing may possibly cause excessive thinning of the blood and an alteration of blood measurement values.

With approval from your doctor, you can start grounding minimally, with perhaps a barefoot walk in the park or sitting barefoot in a grassy yard for an hour or so, or while watching TV in contact with an indoor Earthing product.

Monitor blood frequently in the beginning to determine, under your physician's supervision, whether the medication dosage may be adjusted.

Earthing exposure can be increased gradually but with careful monitoring.

grounded. But I wasn't grounded that time, and the chest pain continued for the following two days when I took two small hikes. I came back home the next day with the pain still there. So I lay down on a grounded bed mat and napped for about a half hour. When I got up, the chest pain was gone completely. I even took a one-hour moderate bike ride afterward without any chest pain. So after chest pain for three days straight, I was greatly relieved.

"I haven't had chest pain since that time or any sign of a-fib since October of 2008, about the time that the financial markets went sour. Anytime I feel anxiety, or periodic fast or irregular heartbeats, I ground myself and thirty minutes later, everything is back to normal. Obviously I'm thrilled to have gone through the tough and anxious times without incident."

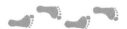

Paul Dunn, Clinton, New York, retired broadcast executive: "I've been in overall excellent health and even walk eighteen holes of golf daily in the summer. But since about 2005, I've had a-fib. For a while each episode would last three or four hours and go away after resting. I experienced skipped beats and felt very tired and sometimes weak.

"Then, the episodes became more frequent, and around 2008 my cardiologist prescribed different medications, including, initially, Coumadin, but later a newer blood thinner. Whether or not they lengthened the time between episodes I have no idea, but they certainly were not very effective. By 2012, I was developing episodes every couple of weeks that would last two to three days. I never knew what triggered them. I have little stress in my life. My doctor was considering a cardiac ablation, a procedure that can correct heart rhythm problems.

"In late 2012, my wife read about Earthing. I was totally skeptical, but in the interest of marital harmony agreed to try it. In mid-December, I was feeling so lousy that she had to drive me to a luncheon meeting. On December 14, I was clearly having an episode. That same night we slept on an Earthing sheet for the first time.

"The next day I was fine. I attributed it to the episode being over. As always, once the heart began beating regularly, usually in the low to mid-60s, I felt fine and could walk rapidly and climb stairs.

"In the twelve months since, I have not had a single episode! This was also confirmed by my cardiologist's technician, who has read my EKGs that are constantly recorded by an implanted device. My doctor has been bemused, but I've told him the sheet is either a wonderful placebo or it really works and I'm not stopping its use."

PROMOTING THE BODY'S ENERGY FUEL—ATP

As a metabolic cardiologist keenly interested in optimizing the energy production of the heart and body, Earthing appears to offer yet another significant benefit as a simple, safe, and effective energy booster.

For years, I have recommended nutritional supplements such as coenzyme Q_{10} (CoQ_{10}), L-carnitine, D-ribose, and magnesium to elevate the bioenergetics of nutrient-starved heart cells and protect them from the ravages of aging, environmental toxins, stress, and relentless oxidation. I have written books and articles about these supplements I refer to as "the awesome foursome." They provide critical raw materials typically deficient in patients. This nutritional approach has worked remarkably and consistently well in helping to restore the failing pumping capacity of sick hearts.

Now, Earthing provides another primary source for cellular restoration and cardiac rehabilitation. One likely venue for such bioelectrical boosting, I believe, is the mitochondria of our trillions of cells. The mitochondria are like microscopic power plants. There can be thousands of them in each cell, depending on how much energy the cell has to provide (heart and kidney cells contain the most). Inside the mitochondria, a complex process goes on nonstop. Electrons are passed along, like a football, through an assembly line of enzymes that create a substance called adenosine triphosphate (ATP), the basic fuel that powers cells to function and repair themselves. By infusing the body with electrons, grounding may ensure an ample supply to mitochondria and may thus contribute to the production of ATP in all cells.

It's taken me most of my cardiology career to learn that the heart is all about ATP, and that effective healing treatment of any form of cardiovascular disease requires the restoration of the heart's ATP production. I've come to realize that sick hearts leak out and lose vital ATP. Cardiac conditions such as angina, heart failure, silent ischemia, and diastolic dysfunction can all cause an ATP deficit.

Another aspect of cellular energy production is that the electrons transported through the assembly line are of a higher energy type, more like a "hot potato" than a football, and that this energy is transferred to ATP. Scientists say these energized electrons are in an "excited state." The electrons provided by the Earth may be of that type—electrons brimming with higher energy. The Earth may thus provide us not only more electrons but supercharged electrons at that!

THE BOTTOM LINE

Like any new idea with the potential to affect health, Earthing needs to be thoroughly studied, tested objectively, and the findings published. I repeatedly submitted our zeta-potential study to mainstream cardiology journals and received not the slightest interest. It is always disappointing to me when conventional medicine rejects new ideas that don't fit into the existing paradigm. Ultimately, if doctors are not exposed to new ideas and opinions, it is the patients who lose out.

Earthing is too good, too natural, and too profound to be ignored.

For sure, in this age of off-the-chart medical costs and skyrocketing chronic disease, medical systems and the doctors working in them need as much help and relief as possible to give patients the most effective and cost-effective care. Earthing offers such a solution and hopefully the medical community will embrace it as more science is produced. It is perhaps the most natural prescription we can recommend to any patient—a perfectly natural adjunct to any clinical strategy.

CHAPTER 12

The Head-to-Toe Connection: Earthing's Systemic Impact

Earthing generates top-to-bottom effects throughout the body. They are often felt dramatically and rapidly, and other times subtly and gradually. In this chapter, you will find a sampling of effects, as related by doctors and patients, illustrating the broad and significant potential of Earthing to improve health.

EARTHING AMBASSADORS

Many people who ground themselves become "Earthing ambassadors" eager to share the news with friends and family. One long-time enthusiast is Jim Healy, a leading pioneer in the research, development, and distribution of cutting-edge monitoring, diagnostic, and therapeutic technologies used by doctors and hospitals. Years ago, he participated in designing the first 911 paramedic rescue vehicles and helicopters. He is chairman of Lead-Lok Corp., an international medical products company headquartered in Sandpoint, Idaho. Here is his Earthing story.

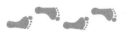

"I've been in the medical instrumentation field for a half-century. In the late 1960s, I started a company specializing in the inspection and upgrading of electrical equipment in hospitals to ensure that the equipment was properly grounded. If not, disturbances or spikes in the electrical current might create a life-threatening shock in a patient connected to a piece of equipment. It was all about grounding the equipment to prevent potential shock. Nobody ever thought that directly grounding a patient could be beneficial.

"When I first heard about Earthing, it made real sense to somebody like me. Clint Ober demonstrated the concept by putting a grounded electrode patch on my leg. The leg was chronically achy. Within twenty minutes, it felt much better. I then started sleeping grounded. I noticed quickly that I slept better, and all the aches and pains that come with aging improved as well.

"I then began to think of how I could help people close to me. One person I thought of was a friend's daughter with multiple sclerosis. The results she got from sleeping grounded were unbelievable. She told me she was now able to get up in the morning without her usual aches and pains.

"Some time afterward she came over to see me. She had been on vacation for a month. She said she hadn't taken her grounded sheet with her and was still feeling great, saying, 'as good or better than before when I was sleeping on it.' Now, back at home and sleeping on the grounded sheet again, she wasn't feeling any difference. She wasn't sure the sheet was working anymore.

"I was curious. I asked where she went on vacation. She and her boyfriend had rented a cottage on the beach in Baja California. For most of the month she never wore shoes. She walked on the sand. She went swimming and snorkeling.

"'That's the whole point,' I told her. 'You *were* grounding yourself every day. Walking barefoot on the Earth. Swimming in saltwater. That's super grounding. There is nothing magical about the grounded sheet or connected to a wall plug or ground rod. It is all about reconnecting to the Earth one way or another. You get the same effect barefoot on the beach or in the park or your backyard garden or sleeping on a grounded sheet. The more hours, the better.'

"She then wanted to know if Earthing might help her mother who had painful rheumatoid arthritis, particularly in the knees. Her mother took two Advils every morning and then would wait an hour or so until they went to work in her body before finally getting out of bed. Otherwise her legs hurt too much.

"I heard back that after a couple of days of sleeping grounded, her mother wasn't taking the pills anymore. She was getting up in the morning without pain, and needless to say was very happy about it. Now, her husband, who was my friend, is a medical professional and a real skeptic. He was observing all this and seeing how it had helped his wife and daughter. He was very surprised about their improvement and then reluctantly told me his own story. He had had a bad left shoulder for years and because of the pain only slept on his right side. After sleeping for a while on the grounded sheet that his wife had put on the bed, he noticed that he was now sleeping on his left side without any pain.

"Then there's the story of an acupuncturist in town. One day, she and I were talking. She said she hadn't been riding her bicycle lately because of pain in one foot. She had treated herself but hadn't gotten any relief. So I gave her some electrode patches with a ground connection and said to give it a try. The following day she called all excited. She couldn't believe it. Her pain was gone. So she then invited some of her patients to sit grounded for a half hour with an electrode patch attached to wherever they had pain. She wasn't charging them for it. The women were coming in three times a week, sitting there, and getting pain relief. I told the acupuncturist that if they would just walk barefoot in their gardens for the same amount of time they would get the same results as they would in her office.

"I also gave a sheet to one of my company directors, a man who suffers with multiple sclerosis. He was also a skeptic. I asked him about it a couple of weeks later and he shrugged it off, saying he gave the sheet to his daughter who has some aches and pains. He said he felt he was too far gone to get any help. A week later, he said his daughter had given it back to him and he decided to try it anyway. He had slept with it for three or four nights. Much of his pain was gone. He was walking better. His legs didn't collapse as often. He still has MS, but his symptoms are greatly reduced. He walks without as much pain and is much more comfortable."

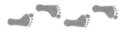

"I Wouldn't Go Anywhere Without My Sheets": Another Earthing ambassador is Donna Tisdale, a top Nashville real estate broker.

"Where do I start?" she said when asked about her Earthing experience.

"Let me start with allergies. I have been plagued with miserable seasonal allergies all my life. As a real estate professional, I'd be out showing property, and I would sneeze maybe ten or fifteen times in a row. I would laugh and tell my clients I'm allergic to the months of May and September. I would buy a giant-sized box of allergy medicine and take it for those entire months. Well, it's been five years now, and the Mays and Septembers have come and gone, and I haven't had to take a single pill in all this time. And I no longer have hidden inflammation in my sinus cavity that reacts to the nasty pollen. So no allergic reactions at all! I've sneezed maybe a few times and that's it. I have not gotten up one single solitary time in the middle of the night to clear my sinuses so I could breathe and sleep! This has been unbelievable.

"For almost twenty years, I had a weird autoimmune skin disease called granuloma annulare. It produced unsightly breakouts on my legs, arms, and trunk. Now it's almost completely gone on my arms, and almost completely gone on my legs. It's amazing. I've been to dermatologists all over the place, and nobody has a cure for it or knows what causes it.

"My ninety-two-year-old mother was incontinent for twenty years. She had bladder surgery, and it didn't work. So she would use fifteen to twenty pads a day. She came to visit for a month about six weeks after she started to sleep grounded. She was using maybe one or two pads a day. 'I think it's the sheets,' she said. She was right. The sheets enabled her to regain control.

"She also had shoulder pain for three years from an injury and could not raise her right hand over her shoulder. One day during her visit I saw her combing her hair with her right hand. I asked her about it. She said, 'My shoulder doesn't hurt anymore. I think it's the sheets.'

"Prior to Earthing, the doctors were telling my husband, Bill, that he would need knee replacement surgery. They were giving him injections into the knee for the pain. Then we started Earthing and he was soon able to stop the injections. A year later, in 2009, he was up and dancing at a family wedding. We hadn't danced together for years because of his knees. His knees are seventy-plus years but they have been doing great since grounding. He hasn't needed the surgery. Previously, he also suffered with plantar fasciitis, and now that's gone, too.

"One of my sisters had that as well. I got her to start Earthing and she got relief as well. Another sister with aggressive rheumatoid arthritis was also helped. A dear friend with Lyme disease experienced as many as fifteen migraines a month. After starting Earthing, she had only one or two a month.

"From the start, we slept much better on the grounded sheets. Bill stopped getting up three times at night like he used to do. A few weeks after we started sleeping grounded, we headed off on a weekend trip out-of-state to visit family. I wanted to take the sheets. Bill didn't. I gave in. Well, he flipped and he flopped at night. He was up. He was down. He didn't sleep well. So when we went to Austin to see the grandchildren for Christmas, guess what? We took the sheets! We slept well. Now we don't go anywhere without them."

THE MOST BENEFITS FOR THE LEAST AMOUNT OF WORK

David Wolfe, San Diego, speaker and author on healthy lifestyle: "Personally, I've seen three surprising changes after I started Earthing six years ago. The first was the disappearance of a stubborn remnant of an infection—likely one of those antibiotic-resistant staph infections. I developed the infection on my big toe about eight years ago and battled it for a couple of years, down to one lump that looked like scar tissue. Occasionally, it would bother me. I used all the healing tools at my disposal and even asked for help from some health professionals I know. But I couldn't eliminate it. Then I started using a grounded floor pad as I worked on my computer or on the telephone. Within two days, the lump was gone. Like magic.

"Similarly, I had a very sensitive tooth for about thirty years. I had cracked it at age fourteen. The tooth was sensitive to cold water and any kind of sugar or sweetener. If I chewed down on a small, hard object like a seed and it pressed against the tooth, there would be a jolt of pain. After a few months of Earthing, I noticed the sensitivity disappeared.

"The biggest change healthwise has been with my allergies. As a kid, they were completely disruptive. I was extremely sensitive to cats and pollen, especially ragweed. Exposure could incapacitate me for two or three days. In pollen season, my lungs would fill with mucus and fluid. I would get intense itchiness in my eyes, ears, and back of the throat. My eyes would tear. The allergies have gotten better over the years as I have improved my nutrition. But Earthing has been like the coup de grace. I've gone through two pollen allergy seasons now without any problem. No symptoms. If I go into a house now where a cat resides, I am good for about an hour. Before I couldn't even go into the house.

"Besides the changes in me, I have seen and heard pretty amazing things when other people are grounded. One woman who came to one of my health seminars was in obvious pain. She was sitting in the front row, and I could see her discomfort written on her face. I went over and asked her about it. She said she suffered with back pain for twenty years. I had a grounding pad with me. I connected it into a wall outlet and she put it inside her blouse against her back. An hour and twenty minutes later, when I finished my talk, her face had totally changed. She couldn't believe what had happened. She said her pain was gone. I was shocked. Everybody in the room was shocked.

"Pretty much everybody who sleeps grounded says they sleep better. One interesting feedback I've gotten from a number of people is that they feel different when they work grounded at their computers. They describe the feeling with words like 'comfort,' 'security,' and 'safety.' A few of them have said they actually don't like working at a computer anymore unless they are grounded.

"In my work as a health educator and speaker, I focus on what's natural, good for healing, and good for people in general. I'm also very much attuned to what is the least amount of work that somebody can do and get the most benefits. That's a number one consideration for me because in the health world people want to get the most benefits for the least amount of work. Well, it became clear to me after about a month of Earthing that this was it. Earthing gives you the most benefits for the least amount of work of anything I've ever seen. There is no work!"

WHAT HEALTH PROFESSIONALS SAY . . .

Improving the Life of a Doctor and His Patients

David Gersten, M.D., Encinitas, California, practitioner of nutritional medicine and integrative psychiatry: "A few years ago, I developed what I called a 'cause and effect' health map that plots out why people get sick with chronic illness and stay sick. I narrowed it down to a simple three-step process. In all chronic illness, you have primary causes (level one), which include genetics, infections, toxins, digestive problems, malabsorption, and mental, emotional, and stress factors. Level two involves reactions to these primary causes, namely through inflammation and the stress response. Level three relates to total body disturbances of biochemistry, or what I call metabolic chaos. Over time, it has become clear to me that Earthing has a profound healing effect on level two.

"I've been grounded for about seven years, and now it's completely integrated into my practice. I see people all the time who come to a doctor like me as a last resort. The first feedback I usually hear after a patient starts Earthing is an e-mail the following morning that says, 'I just had the best sleep in many years.'

"I provided a grounding unit to a ninety-six-year-old friend who had severe osteoarthritis for probably twenty-five years. I didn't explain a word to her. I just explained it to her son. After a few days, I called to see how she was doing. He said his mother, a well-known folk medicine healer in San Diego for decades, told him her pain was down more than three-quarters. But what was really amazing was that her passion for life had come back. She had had a stroke six months before, and, although she recovered from the physical effects, she had lost her typical passion for life. This was a vital woman who was still traveling and giving lectures. 'It's back,' her son told me.

"I see many patients with chronic fatigue syndrome (CFS), a problem that often involves cognitive issues like memory, concentration, focus, and brain fog. One such patient was a sixty-five-year-old woman. She also had hypertension for a very long time. I told her to get grounded. On day thirty-one after she started, she e-mailed me to say that not only was her energy much improved but that her cognition had also suddenly returned. Moreover, her blood pressure numbers had dropped and were normalizing. I advised her to monitor her blood pressure carefully each day. She had been taking two blood pressure medications that another doctor had prescribed. Her blood pressure came down so fast that she was now able to take a much weaker prescription, and still maintain a normal blood pressure. Her fatigue and most of her other CFS symptoms vastly improved.

"Another CFS patient suffered with anxiety. Immediately after she grounded herself, she had a significant improvement in her anxiety, overall health, and energy. She described a sense of renewed connectedness to the Earth, to others around her, and to the absolute core of her being. She felt this connectedness so much when she was grounded that she took her bed pad with her to work. She slept on it at night and used it at her desk during the day. She said she was experiencing her deepest self, 'a new me,' she called it, without all the worry, the fear, the anxiety, and the restless mind. 'I'm changed at the core,' she said.

"The feedback I have from patients is now so strong that I know predictably, as a doctor, this will change a person's life. Maybe three out of nearly one hundred patients have said they didn't notice any difference.

"In terms of my own personal experiences, I didn't see anything miraculous, at least not for a while. For decades, I have suffered with keratoconus, a condition in which the cornea of the eye becomes progressively thin, blows out like a balloon, leading to significant visual loss. You can't get a contact to fit anymore. I've had five corneal transplants over the years. Three in the right eye were rejected, resulting in considerable inflammation and the formation of hundreds of minute blisters on the surface of the cornea. In the latter stages of rejection, the pain is absolutely agonizing. I often needed to use huge doses of Tylenol with codeine. Moreover, I would wake up each morning with drainage coming out of the eye.

"It was a good year and a half into the rejection of my 2004 transplant when I began to ground myself. In addition to the pain, I was waking up each morning with drainage coming out of the eye. After about four months, I realized that the drainage was not there. From that day on, there has been no drainage at all. The pain level has stayed low, and it's very tolerable almost all the time. Very seldom do I require a strong painkiller. But now I'm seven years into a rejection that would not have been bearable without Earthing.

"In any case, I have no vision out of the right eye. Although I haven't had the corneal transplant rejection issue with the left eye, I was definitely losing vision in that eye and was quite concerned to say the least. I had been going downhill for about fifteen years until I started Earthing. Then the vision loss stopped and reversed. My optometrist was amazed at the dramatic improvement in vision and said he has never seen anyone who had a degenerative eye disease that suddenly reversed after decades. For me, this was pretty miraculous.

"Another personal experience made me keenly aware of the power of Earthing. I was working at night in a clinic and had stepped outside to take a short break. While outside, I walked smack into a metal post with a 'No Parking' sign. The side of the post was like a dull knife blade, and it put a half-inch gash in my forehead down to the bone. It was bleeding badly. I ran back into the clinic and had my nurse clean the wound and bandage it up. I would have sent any patient with this kind of cut to the emergency room. But I had more patients to see. The next day, I pulled off the bandages and there was just a small line, like a small surgical incision, where the cut was. There was no sign of redness, heat, swelling, or pain. There was virtually no inflammation. On day two, I could just make out the edges of the gash. The edges of the cut were starting to come together and heal. On day six, it was completely healed without any sign of the cut at all."

Less Pain, Better Mobility, More Energy

R. J. Wilson, M.B., Ch.B., FRACGP, Peregian Beach, Australia, general practitioner: "My appreciation of Earthing comes from analyzing the reasons for my own, and my wife's health and vitality. Before coming to Australia, we spent much time grounded either in the sea or through walking barefoot and gardening in New Zealand and England. The Queensland climate in Australia offered far more opportunity to get more of it.

"Our levels of energy increased. Our robust immune systems meant a lot less bouts of infection and, specifically my wife, who coped with a severely arthritic ankle joint from a fracture dislocation sustained while skiing in 1986, reported much reduced levels of inflammation, stiffness, swelling, and pain. Initially, I attributed our new found levels of health to more fresh sea air, seawater cleansing swims/surfs, sunlight, and healthier eating. But there was more to it. It was the Earth's influence as well.

"I advised arthritic and chronic pain patients to get as much outside barefoot time as possible. When they did, they reported fewer symptoms and improved mobility and energy with less reliance on drugs for these symptoms. The responses seemed much better in the summer months when climatic warmth encouraged more outdoor barefoot time.

"Recently I discovered the research behind the 'Earthing process.' Particularly fascinating to me as a doctor is the theory of the Earth's influence on inflammation. This inspired me to be Earthed as much as possible, both out-side and inside. By stumbling across this ancient wisdom and new research, I have at my disposal a simple application at little or no cost to recommend to patients as part of their journey to optimal wellness, thereby reducing their reliance on pharmaceuticals and costly alternative therapies."

Shifting Lives with Earthing—A Psychiatrist's Perspective

Tracy Latz, M.D., Mooresville, North Carolina, integrative psychiatry: "I love digging in the dirt and feeling my connection to the Earth. I find walking barefoot in the grass to be a great stress reducer. In my psychi-atric practice, I often recommend Earthing to patients as part of an inte-grative approach to healing. As a physician, I consider it to be a powerful tool in my multidimensional healing medicine bag.

"Some patients are open to the concept of Earthing; others aren't. Some will say, 'I don't have enough time to stand or walk outside barefoot' or 'I don't want to pay for an Earthing mat or sheet.' Patients who ground them-selves, dozens of them now, tend to feel much better as a result. They are individuals with different emotional, mental, and physical problems, and often combinations of problems.

"They often say they sleep much better. This is a big deal for many of my patients.

"I have observed Earthing helping psychiatric patients in the following ways:

"For those with anxiety (post-traumatic stress, generalized anxiety, panic disorder, etc.), it generates an improved sense of safety. By improving sleep, Earthing can help normalize serotonin levels in the brain as it decreases cortisol (an anxiety-inducing hormone). When cortisol levels are high, there is a tendency to go into 'fight-or-flight'/panic responses to stressful situations and to become more easily angered or irritable. As cortisol lev-els decrease and stabilize, we become more centered, peaceful, and calm. We get more easily into our heart and have more compassion for our self as well as for others. Some patients stop Earthing after their anxiety gets better. I have to remind them about what helped them get better.

"For depression, Earthing can assist with stabilizing serotonin levels as noted above. Serotonin assists with decreasing crying spells, near-tearfulness, and obsessive/repetitive negative thoughts. When depressive symptoms lessen, energy levels rise and tolerance to stressful situations, pain, or discomfort improves.

"Many chronic pain patients, referred to me from pain management doctors, have not responded well to, or are resistant to, taking medication. With Earthing, they often have decreased inflammatory problems overall.

"I've seen significant improvement of gluten intolerance and irritable bowel symptoms. Patients may not be completely cured, but their GI and stomach issues are better. They have less pain and anxiety.

"I recommend Earthing for autoimmune conditions. Two patients with systemic lupus erythematosis are doing much better. Their primary doctors attribute their improvement to 'a calm period' in their disease process.

"I see many patients with chronic fatigue, people who have exhausted their adrenal hormones. Most of them have a history of intense stress. With Earthing, they are much less fatigued and calmer. As their sleep cycle improves, the adrenal issues start improving. They have more energy; they feel better.

"One of my friends is a computer systems programmer for a major nationwide bank. He works with multiple computer screens for up to ten hours a day six or seven days per week. He is always under pressure answering SOS calls and fixing this or that glitch. He hardly has time to relax and the pace was wearing him down and aging him at an alarming rate. One day I brought him an Earthing mat. I told him to place it under his bare feet at his desk since that's where he spends the biggest chunk of his time.

"He called the next day to tell me he loves his 'fizzy feet.'

"'Fizzy feet?'

"'Yeah, I can feel the fizzies in my feet and coming up my legs,' he explained. 'I really feel good for the first time in a long time. And I slept so well.'

"My friend is sticking with it, enjoying his 'fizzies' and feeling good.

"Personally, I immediately slept more soundly after I started grounding in 2011. I also experienced much less pain in my left knee that had been intermittently bothering me for a dozen years after I chipped a divot of bone out of my femur in a freak accident. Now I only get rare slight twinges when the weather gets real cold suddenly or there are abrupt changes in atmospheric pressure.

"I sent my mother an Earthing sheet for her chronic pain and fibro-myalgia-like symptoms. She was soon able to work in the garden for the first time in three years. She now sleeps through the night, which she wasn't doing before. She can walk down stairs better now.

"My three teenagers sleep grounded. My eldest is a musician and had previously complained about chronic neck and shoulder muscle tension during marching band or indoor drumline competitions. My two sons are athletes—playing high school football and lacrosse. They all say they rest better, have less muscle inflammation, and more rapid recovery from injuries since Earthing."

A New, Powerful, Anti-Inflammatory Tool

Martin Gallagher, M.D., D.C., Jeannette, Pennsylvania, medical doctor and chiropractor: "There are many tools that integrative doctors like me have at hand to reduce inflammation and promote healing. We now have another: Earthing. Hitherto unknown and overlooked, it is rapidly emerging as a natural, simple, powerful, and essential antidote. In my own practice, it neatly supports and enhances other modalities that include medication, chiropractic, prolotherapy, acupuncture, diet change, oral and IV vitamin therapies, and meditation.

"Earthing has become a key recommendation I make to patients. I've observed therapeutic benefits among individuals with acute and chronic pain, fibromyalgia, migraine headaches, chronic tendinitis, bursitis, and arthritis. Many of the autoimmune disorders, including rheumatoid arthritis and lupus, can be modulated by grounding.

"Depression, insomnia, and anxiety are common among chronic pain patients. Earthing is a unique drugless method that helps to downregulate pain, spasm, and inflammation, while simultaneously promoting deeper, restful sleep. These factors help people in distress to recover much more effectively and quickly.

"I've had patients with chronic hip, leg, or shoulder pain who were taking anti-inflammatory drugs. When rolling over in bed at night, they would get a jolt of pain and wake up. Now, with Earthing, they sleep more soundly and don't wake up as frequently. Earthing has, in fact, consistently helped patients with insomnia issues."

TMJ, Bruxism, Gum Disease Helped by Earthing

Chuck Munier, D.M.D., Augusta, Maine, general dentistry: "I was trained as a mechanical engineer before dentistry and take an engineer's show-me attitude to new things. Earthing was brought to my attention by an enthusiastic patient. I was naturally skeptical. However, one night of sleeping on an Earthing sheet eliminated my skepticism.

"I had been suffering for a few years with a chronic foot infection unresponsive to repeated medication. After one night grounded, I noticed a healing process underway. After one week, the infection was gone. Now, almost three years later, it has never returned. This was truly remarkable.

"I have been treating dental patients for forty years and have learned to manage inflammation as a key to avoiding and minimizing disease. Earthing adds an electrical approach to the dietary, lifestyle, and exercise model that I have used to address inflammation.

"Earthing effectively helps relieve patients with acute temporomandibular joint (TMJ) or jaw pain, bruxism (teeth clenching and grinding), sinus issues, headaches, and sleeping and snoring problems. An Earthing patch placed directly over the offending joint often rapidly reduces acute TMJ symptoms. Chronic problems take longer to respond.

"Periodontal (gum) disease is an inflammatory process that can be helped by anti-inflammatory medications. It responds as well to Earthing, which seems to limit inflammation in the body, and in so doing aids in the restoration of healthy gums."

Conditions Often Heal That Typically Never Get Better

Wendy Menigoz, D.N., Bourbonnais, Illinois, neuromyologist and pain specialist: "When I first heard about Earthing several years ago, I immediately got my husband grounded. He was suffering dreadfully from severe leptospirosis, a bacterial infection that can lead to death. He had lost considerable weight, his kidneys were failing, and his blood pressure was highly elevated. He had hardly slept in three weeks. The doctors told me they had done everything in their power and didn't think he would survive.

"As soon as he was grounded, he fell asleep deeply. When he awoke, he got up with energy that I hadn't seen in months. He continued sleeping well and gradually got his strength and weight back. His health dramatically improved and his doctors were dumbfounded.

"My husband's healing experience inspired me to introduce Earthing to my patients. The results have been remarkable. I've repeatedly seen conditions healed or improved that typically never get better, or that are typically treated with medication simply to manage the symptoms.

"Patients have told me that headaches have disappeared or dramatically lessened in intensity. Several women with multiple sclerosis have had remarkable remissions. One of them is a woman whose developmentally disabled daughter also benefitted with major relief of arthritic ankles. Patients with sciatica, plantar fasciitis, and various kinds of diabetic neuropathy have also benefitted. They take much less pain medication. They feel better and they are happier.

"One man had been scheduled for double knee-replacement surgery. His pain level dropped so much in a short period of time that the operation was put on hold. He's out biking and exercising. He couldn't do that before.

"I told a friend about Earthing whose husband is a veterinarian with chronic hip pain. She brought him a grounding mat and he said he would use 'the silly thing' to humor her. He put it in his bed. The next morning he woke up without pain. The pain is still gone two years later!

"I've seen many cases of improved blood pressure. A few male patients mentioned improvement of erectile dysfunction, which I assume is a result of better circulation.

"Some patients, after experiencing significant benefits from Earthing, have asked me, 'How long do I have to do this?' I laugh, and answer that for as long as they want to feel better."

Speeds Pain Relief, Bolsters Bodywork

Many bodyworkers have told us that sleeping and working grounded has made a big difference in their energy level and endurance, and that their clients feel the difference as well.

Tina Michaud-Gray, R.N., L.M.T., Dover, New Hampshire, pain specialist: "I've worked for twenty years with soft tissue injury, and acute and chronic pain. My focus is reestablishing pain-free range of motion, muscular flexibility, and strength after injury or surgery. Doctors are surprised at the rate of healing, restored function, and tissue repair when I use one or a combination of the technologies. All of them on their own can create a higher level of repair and healing, and Earthing is one of the best tools I have. As an example, we treated a sixty-six-year-old woman who had a facelift. She was off pain medication in thirty-six hours and experienced accelerated healing so that a week later there was no sign of surgical bruising.

"Ever since I started sleeping and working grounded more than ten years ago, everything changed for me. I put an Earthing mat under my massage table that allows me to double the amount of massages I can do without wearing myself out. Before Earthing I was doing five to six hour massages a day, but I was exhausted afterward, sometimes so much so that I could hardly grip the steering wheel of my car on the drive home. The day after I started Earthing I did eleven massages. I routinely have days of eight or nine without my hands burning out as before and without having to recover afterward. I have plenty of energy.

"In my bodywork practice, I have also developed a technique using Earthing patches to dissolve knots and trigger points that allows me to do many things at once, from antiaging facials to pain relief."

Relief from Burns

Over the years we have observed that Earthing rapidly reduces the pain and aftereffects of burns. In the following story, Earthing mats were applied directly to burn sites. Earthing patches can also be applied adjacent to a burn.

Louis Gordon, B.Ac., Toowoomba, Queensland, Australia, acupuncturist: "Over the years I have seen and treated many serious burns. I am aware that if cold water is applied immediately for about thirty minutes, the damage from severe deep burns can be reduced. Applying copious amounts of fresh aloe vera to burns is also beneficial. From my personal experience, however, blisters still form and last for many days to weeks, and redness persists for many days as well.

"While cooking a meal for friends in 2012, I suffered severe burns to my right hand, face, ear, and back of the head from boiling fat. As soon as I overcame the shock from the accident, I bathed the burned areas with cold water for about a half hour and then squeezed aloe vera sap onto my damaged skin. Blisters were already forming.

"I now pulled out two Earthing mats. I placed one around my hand and wrist, covering the burn areas. I pressed the other against the affected areas on my ear and head. I felt a very strong tingling sensation on the burn sites.

"I sat down and tried to relax for a while. My wife checked in on me about twenty minutes later. I took off the mats. We were both stunned, as were our dinner guests. The redness was nearly gone! The blisters had essentially retracted and were also nearly gone.

"During the meal, I kept rotating a pad from one site to the other. After the meal, we retired early. I told my wife I would probably have to cancel patients for a few days because the burns on my fingers were exactly where I insert acupuncture needles.

"I slept grounded and slept soundly. In the morning, to my amazement, there was absolutely no redness and the blisters were nonexistent. I went to work and it was business as usual. It may be a good idea for every first aid kit to contain an Earthing mat of some size.

"I have been an acupuncturist for more than thirty years and each month insert over 3,000 acupuncture needles. As a result of this activity, I developed a repetitive strain injury in my right shoulder. The pain was about 4 out of 10 most of the time, (10 being extremely painful). At the close of my workday, the pain would rise to a 7–8 level, with the rhomboid muscle starting to spasm. After five weeks of Earthing (using a mat daily when at the computer and while watching television, and sleeping grounded nightly), the shoulder pain dropped to about a 1–2 level generally and at the end of the day never above 4. In addition, my sleep is serene."

THE ANTIAGING CONNECTION

Growing older is inevitable. Antiaging strategies are not about living to 100 or 120, but about growing older gracefully and with energy. The goal is to prevent and minimize illness and to develop physical and mental potential in the pursuit of satisfaction and aliveness. Can Earthing help the process? We sure think so!

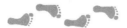

Arvord Belden, Ph.D., Yountville, California, retired clinical psychologist: "I've been sleeping grounded pretty regularly for more than a dozen years. Within a year, I realized that I wasn't going to doctors like I used to do. My hands and hip hurt me less from arthritis. I also noticed that my mind seemed to be clearer, and I had more energy and stamina.

"After a year, I had a checkup with my doctor, and he was amazed at my excellent health given my age.

"Now after all these years of continued Earthing, I can't say I've reversed the aging process. I still have the arthritis, but I don't need to take any medication for it. In fact, I don't take a single medication for anything. I feel darn good for somebody in his nineties. My energy is good.

"I used to do a lot of yard work, including tree pruning, and I had my share of cuts, scrapes, and even falls. A few years ago, I was out on my recumbent three-wheeler bike and I took a fall. I banged myself up but didn't break anything, and I healed up nice and quick. Same thing with the yard work.

"My sleep improved after I started this. If I wake up at night, it seems like after a minute or so, I am back sleeping again."

MULTIPLE BENEFITS—
THE HOLISTIC IMPACT OF EARTHING

People who start Earthing because of a sleep or a pain problem are often surprised to experience a broad array of relief. Here are a few such stories:

Lynn Deene, Milo, Michigan, retired medical practice administrator: "In 2010 I started Earthing looking for relief for bilateral swollen and painful Achilles tendons and plantar fasciitis. For over a year, I had tried exercise, ice packs, massage, and physical therapy, with little or no relief.

"At the end of each day, my calves and feet were painful. Every step was torture, no matter how active or inactive the day. Getting out of bed in the morning, it felt like I was standing on blocks of wood. It took several slow steps to loosen up my feet.

"I also had left shoulder and upper arm pain from a fall six months earlier. I experienced minimum relief from therapy, pain relievers, and stretching exercises.

"I dealt with urinary frequency, headaches, fatigue that sleep didn't relieve, other muscle aches, and a feeling of heaviness in my legs that came after a few minutes of my daily walks, and chronic knee pain from a twenty-year-old injury caused from a horse kick.

"I took hypertension medication daily.

"I have led a healthy lifestyle all my life—no alcohol, no tobacco, eat well, drink lots of water, take supplements, have regular adjustments, do daily exercise, and love the outdoors.

"I read about Earthing and got myself an Earthing mat. I put it on the floor at my computer. After a ten-hour day at the computer, I noticed that I didn't get my usual headache after a few hours and I wasn't nearly as fatigued at the end of the work day. I had more energy for my after-work walk.

"I was so excited that I got a half sheet for our bed. My husband was willing to give it a try.

"After two weeks I noticed less muscle pain. After three weeks, my Achilles tendons were less swollen and didn't hurt at the end of the day. After four months, I was like a new person. My tendons felt normal. The fasciitis was completely gone. The knee pain, 'creakiness,' and heaviness in my legs were gone. My mobility became stronger, quicker, more flexible. I wasn't fatigued at 10 AM, as before.

"The shoulder and arm pain was greatly relieved. The urinary symptoms were gone. I didn't have to plan my life around bathroom availability. I was able to lower my blood pressure medication—from 20 to 5 milligrams—with a consistently lower reading that I haven't seen since I started on medication more than a dozen years ago.

"My husband has also benefited. He has had very little muscle pain, sleeps more soundly, and with less snoring, and has more energy during the day.

"Looking back more than three years later, could I ever have possibly believed that my pain, fatigue, and incontinence would be gone? The best that I had hoped for was some relief from tendon pain. I was really afraid my active life was going to be severely compromised. Instead, I am able to enjoy more and do more physically."

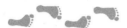

Graeme Dalton, London, artist/designer: "I've had relief from some twenty years of insomnia (since I was about sixteen!) and eczema. I had tried all the usual kinds of treatments for these problems. Either they wouldn't work at all or just would work temporarily.

"I started going barefoot in a nearby park for an hour a day in 2012. I couldn't believe it, but the insomnia simply vanished! I was astounded. I was in bed before midnight and waking up at 7:30 feeling great and full of energy. The skin rashes I had for years cleared up and almost disappeared.

"Psychologically, I feel much better than in years. I'm confident, happy, excited, and less stressed in general.

"My other half had back trouble for a while from dragging around heavy bags and was always in pain and almost half bent over. Now her back pain is almost completely gone.

"Both of us sailed through the cold months without the usual colds, sniffles, and the winter blues.

"As an artist and musician, most of what I do involves creative processes and inspiration. In the last nine months, since starting Earthing, I have created more paintings, taken more photographs, and written more songs than at any one time over the past seven or eight years. The creative juices keep flowing. I credit this to the overall effect of Earthing on the physiological and psychological levels. I seem more balanced in my whole being and more focused on the bigger picture rather than getting carried away with the small details. This has made me happier and more content, which in turn leads to a more creative mind, which leads to more creativity.

"I sleep grounded on a sheet all the time now.

"My experience inspired me to tell friends about Earthing. One suffered from terrible eczema of the hands. She started using a grounded mat

Tale of Two Towns . . .

Fairfield, Iowa (population 9,464)

Fairfield lists some 500 businesses, reportedly more than any other American community its size. It is home to Maharishi University of Management and several thousand meditators. Since 2010, many have incorporated Earthing into their daily lifestyle. Their comments reveal the broad spectrum of Earthing benefits:

- "I suffered with severe pain in my right arm due to many hours working on the computer. After a few days the pain was reduced significantly and doesn't bother me anymore."

- "I have Huntington's disease and involuntary movements. After one month I slept better, bit my tongue less, and swallowed liquids easier."

- "I used to sleep poorly because of the intense pain of rheumatoid arthritis. A month after starting Earthing, I began sleeping better, and over time, deeper and more restful. My wrist and knee joints became less painful, with more mobility. My blood work (SED rate to measure inflammation), always in the 60–90 range, came down and most recently was at 29! This was the first time in five years I have been in the normal range."

- "I was diagnosed with ALS (Lou Gehrig's). My sleep became erratic at best. My sister gave me a grounding sheet, and it really helped! I can easily go back to sleep. I also use a grounding mat at work and feel that this, along with diet, have helped me remain stable for the last year."

- "My intense hot flashes are about 90 percent gone since I started sleeping grounded two months ago."

- "Earthing got rid of my PMS."

- "I am able to sleep and rest better, which has always been a problem because of stress related to traumatic childhood abuse. I am happier."

- "I got an Earthing mat for my thirteen-year-old dog who had had a chronic infection in one eye for a year. I used eye drops, which worked temporarily, but the condition would return. When he started sleeping grounded, the infection cleared up and didn't return."

- "I noticed a profound reduction in chronic anxiety within a month. With less anxiety, my general mood has been more positive and optimistic. I feel happier."

. . . Models for a Healthier World

Haines, Alaska (population 2,500)

Haines, surrounded by breathtaking mountains, glaciers, and waterways, attracts numerous visitors for fishing, hiking, heli-skiing, and, from fall to February, the largest bald eagle concentration in the world. Earthing was introduced in 2012. Here is a sampling of experiences:

- David Olerud suffered a severed spinal column in 1987 when a wall fell on him at a construction site. He was left a paraplegic, wheelchair-bound, and with "a dead lower body," as he puts it. Since he started sleeping grounded, he has experienced improvement in bowel function, increased mobility in the hips and in one leg, and a greater ability to cause muscle contractions down to the knee. After a few months, he began to take some unassisted steps with a walker for the first time since his accident. "These things may not sound like a big deal, but they are a big achievement for somebody in my condition," says Olerud, a man with an inspiring, positive spirit, who leads an active life as the founder of the American Bald Eagle Foundation, a nature education project in Haines.

- Janis and Shane Horton, proprietors of the "Eagle's Nest Motel," put up a sign outside proclaiming "First in Nation: Earthing Room Available." Typical comments from guests, they say, are: "Best sleep I've had in years" or "I woke up and my pain was gone . . . what a surprise."

- Tim Walter, proprietor of Haines Propane and a captain in the local volunteer fire department, suffered with constant pain since 1993 when he ruptured four vertebral discs. That, and a couple of hernias, made "every day a struggle," he says. "I was extremely skeptical about Earthing, but after sleeping grounded a couple of nights, my pain was 90 percent gone. It's been a year now and I am pretty much without pain. I'm still broken up inside, and if I overdo something in my work, and get hurt, I heal very fast."

- Rocky Seward, laborer, and distant relative of William Seward, the secretary of state under Abraham Lincoln and Andrew Johnson who negotiated the purchase of Alaska from Russia in 1867: "I suffered from real bad snoring, like a freight train, and also sleep apnea. I would wake up, choking for breath. I didn't sleep well for years and didn't have good energy. I'm told I don't snore anymore and I'm not bothered with the apnea. I sleep deep. I have plenty of energy during the day. It's been a blessing for me."

at her computer. Unbelievably, within a week, the eczema pretty much cleared up, and she was sleeping and feeling much better.

"Another friend, a man in his midsixties, had problems with his hands all his life. I'm not sure about his condition, but he couldn't make a fist. Over several months, his condition gradually improved and he could pretty much make a fist again.

"It is all truly amazing."

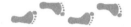

Karen Ball, Beaverton, Oregon, massage therapist: "In 2011, I was in terrible shape. I had been suffering with serious insomnia for twenty-two years, sleeping maybe two to three hours per night. I had digestive difficulties, mild depression, bloating, fifteen years of hot flashes, bone density issues, and severe arthritis and muscle contracture in my right hip that caused pain and restricted movement. To top it off, at 244 pounds, I was 80 pounds overweight.

"Sleeping pills, megadoses of melatonin, antihistamines, supplements, hot baths, herbs, teas, meditation, breathing exercises, relaxation CDs, and so many more things were making little impact on my problems. I tried everything.

"In 2011, I started sleeping grounded. The first three nights I didn't get any sleep, but I had great energy from laying on it seven to nine hours per night. Moreover, I lost considerable inflammation so that my severely swollen ankles now appeared normal. I lost 4.5 pounds of swelling those first three nights! Not real weight loss; just a very noticeable decrease of swelling.

"It took six nights before I got a good night's sleep. But from August 2011 to October 2013, I have had four to eight hours of sleep every night except for maybe a couple of nights. My sleep situation has, in fact, improved to the point where I have been increasingly sleeping through the night for weeks at a time without getting up to pee. Better sleep is a huge deal for me. I can only lose weight when I sleep five hours or more. I have now lost forty pounds, and basically by not doing anything, just sleeping more. I need to lose another forty, and to do that I'll need to stop eating bread when I shouldn't.

"After my ankles, my knees became normal size without swelling. I could actually see my kneecap for the first time in five years. My pain was reduced. The contracture in my right thigh went away. The position of the femur corrected itself, and was no longer pressing against the side of the hip socket. I had greater range of movement, less pain, and for the first time in years, could exercise to reverse the muscle atrophy that had developed over a decade. Walking and other forms of exercise had been very painful. I could now do those things.

"In recent years, my hip pain and restrictions were so bad that at times I couldn't manage more than a four-inch stride. I am a tall woman with long legs yet I was barely able to get my leg over the side of a tub, and had to lift my leg with my hands to get into bed or into a car. Gradually, I've been able to extend my stride to eighteen inches on a good day, and it has been getting better all the time.

"I still walk with a cane most of the time, but when I don't my side-to-side hip sway is less than half of what it was before. The sway increases pain so I use the cane for support and to minimize the sway. My ability to bend my knees has increased. I can cross either leg over center now. I could not before. I can lift things now that before would cause severe hip pain. I have been able to do yard work on my half acre, walk back and forth to the chicken coop, and sometimes log a mile and a half of daily walking. I am working continually to strengthen the weak leg muscles so that maybe one day I will be able to walk without a cane. Meanwhile, it looks as if I am pushing off further into the future a hip replacement I was supposed to have at one time.

"My night sweats stopped, and then my hot flashes diminished, and stopped completely in December 2011. What a relief!

"I hadn't realized how depressed I had been before until I became increasingly aware of a greater sense of well-being and return to health. Although I am aware of my limitations, I can do so much more now. My capacity keeps growing and the improvements continue. For instance, I have been able to pivot on my right foot for the first time in twelve years without any pain anywhere. I can carry forty pound bags of chicken feed. Normally, any kind of weight carried would cause lots of pain.

"Clearly the more time I spend grounded, the better I feel."

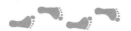

Gaby Buiskool, Linschoten, Netherlands, craniosacral therapist: "In 2012 I heard about Earthing and began walking barefoot outside. I noticed that I became more restful and felt more physically grounded. I also measured the acidity of my urine via pH strips, and found that the strips showed slightly alkaline values (between 7 and 7.4) every time that I went barefoot for at least half an hour. Otherwise, the values measured an average of 6.5, which was not too bad either. I became convinced that the physical contact with the Earth was indeed doing 'something extra.'

"I then started using a conductive mat inside. I put my feet and hands on it and immediately they became warmer. Something happened to the blood flow.

"After two nights sleeping with my bare legs on the mat, the tension in my shoulders disappeared. After a week, there were other changes. My digestion gave fewer problems. I could eat things that I hadn't tolerated for years. My thyroid was normalized. My night sweats stayed away. My skin became softer and less dry, especially my legs.

"I then started using an Earthing sheet. If I am cold, I find I become warmer more quickly with the sheet. I noticed also that during the first two weeks I didn't sleep as well as before. This seemed logical to me. My body went to work solving problems. I compare this experience to a repair or remodeling in your home. Before everything is fine and works well again, you go through a period of clutter and discomfort. After about a month I slept much better and have needed less hours of sleep. I noticed that the varicose veins in my legs became less visible. I am hopeful that they will disappear altogether over time.

"It's been more than a year. I sleep grounded and ground during the day as much as possible. During the cold weather, I didn't go outside barefoot much, and noticed some symptoms come back, although much less intense than before. Other symptoms were simply gone. During the summer I walked barefoot again and that helped my body recover. As a hypersensitive person, it seems that every hour of physical grounding counts.

"With the mat under my feet at my computer, I am able to finish work without physical discomfort, even if it takes several hours. Before I could do computer work for maybe one and a half hours at the most.

In working with clients, I can work more deeply with my feet on an Earthing mat than before."

ALLERGIES

Over the years many people have told us that Earthing helps reduce or eliminate symptoms of common allergies. Here's another example:

Cynthia Fertal, Bethlehem, Pennsylvania, hypnotherapist: "I have had numerous cats in my house through the years. They literally found me, and being the animal lover that I am, they were always welcome, even though I am allergic to them. I can be in the same room with them for just a short period of time, and then I would develop sneezing along with red, itchy, and watery eyes.

"Since sleeping grounded in the latter part of 2012, I have no longer reacted . . . and that happened practically overnight. I have challenged myself by rubbing my face in my cat's fur. And no reaction!

"When out grocery shopping, I used to avoid the laundry detergent aisle at all costs. The smells would assault my senses and I would immediately start to sneeze. If I didn't walk away, my eyes would start to water and my throat felt scratchy. So needless to say, I stayed away from there and ordered my hypoallergenic detergent online. I can't say I enjoy the fragrances of laundry detergents in the stores, but I no longer need to shy away from those aisles. I can now walk through without any ill effects. All these sensitivity/allergy issues disappeared in an extremely short time.

"Moreover, my husband and I are both sleeping better since we started Earthing. My husband frequently used to get up three, four, and even five times during the night to use the bathroom. He now usually sleeps through the night.

"I've also had a major decrease in the frequency of headaches, plus significant improvement in the arthritic pain and swelling of my fingers. I can now make a fist without pain. And if I develop some stiffness in the knees, a night's sleep on the sheet, enables me to get out of bed with a spring in my step. It's nice feeling thirty years younger! I am now quite addicted to feeling good."

ARTHRITIS

The most prevalent form of arthritis is osteoarthritis, also known as degenerative joint disease, wear-and-tear arthritis, or just plain arthritis. The incidence increases with age. Rheumatoid arthritis (RA) differs from osteo in that it is an autoimmune disease, the result of the immune system attacking the body's own tissue. RA can affect other body parts besides joints, such as the eyes, mouth, and lungs. Of these two common forms of arthritis, RA is the most inflammatory. Either one causes pain, stiffness, and can lead to inactivity and disability.

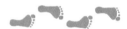

Sheila Curtiss, Draper, Utah, sales: "I was born unhealthy. I'm amazed that I'm alive now. If it weren't for Earthing, I'm not sure I would be.

"I used to have scary episodes of heart fibrillation. They stopped shortly after I started grounding myself and haven't returned. The constant hot flashes I had been experiencing for some years stopped within the first month of grounding.

"But it was the effect on my rheumatoid arthritis that made the biggest and quickest impression on me. I had bad pain and swelling in both knees, particularly the left, and was kind of hobbling all the time. I would have flare-ups from time to time, and, with each episode, it seemed like they were getting worse. The one knee was so swollen I could barely get my leg into my pants. I'd have to lift my leg to get into the car. And all my other joints popped and cracked. Elbows. Wrists. Shoulders. When you hear your joints pop, you wonder what's going on? Am I going to break something?

"I knew one of the top orthopedic surgeons in the area and consulted with him. He told me I should have knee surgery in the next six to eight weeks and until then be careful because my knee could lock up on me. I might fall and hurt myself.

"The following weekend I heard Clint Ober speak at a health conference. His idea sounded interesting to me and I decided to follow up immediately. I got grounded. And in three weeks, the pain and swelling were gone. Gradually, over time all my joints quit popping.

"I've been grounded since 2000, and it has made such a big impact on my health that I stay grounded all the time. People began calling me the bare-foot lady. The only time I'm not grounded is walking from point A to point B, but maybe that will change when they start making grounded shoes.

"Now, years later, I'm doing really well for somebody my age. I walk and exercise, probably not as much as I should, but I'm able to do it without any problem. I walk up and down steps in my house without a problem either. I can move freely. I have become addicted to Earthing. I love the feeling and can tell the difference when I am not grounded."

Steve Garner, West Valley City, Utah, auto technician: "Working on cars for a living is brutal on the hands and body. But that's what I was doing for years until rheumatoid arthritis put me out of action.

"In 1993, I was diagnosed with RA after developing a lot of pain in my hands, ankles, and knees. For the next twelve years, I went to the rheumatology clinic at a university medical center every three months for treatment and evaluation. They put me on six different prescription drugs during that time. Each one had side effects that I couldn't live with.

"One medication I received was called diclofenac. The side effects were terrible: headaches, dizziness, and my guts feeling like they wanted out. I told the doctor that this was not the drug for me. She then prescribed methotrexate but warned me that it could also cause a lot of side effects. It sure did. After about a week, the pain had gone down quite a bit and the inflammation was a little better, but I felt like I had a constant cold with a runny nose, head congestion, and headaches. These were just some of the side effects.

"Meanwhile, my sleep was disturbed from the pain and my performance at work was suffering. The disease was taking the fun and purpose out of life. I began taking massive amounts of ibuprofen, starting with 200 to 500 milligrams (mg) daily. This was just barely taking down the pain and very little of the inflammation. I increased the daily doses to as much as 3,000 mg. I lived like this for five years.

"In 2005, I was forced to retire because of the constant pain and inflammation in my hands. It was impossible to continue my work.

"A couple of years before, I had been given a grounded sheet as a gift, but I was too skeptical. I stashed it in the closet. It sounded too weird to me. After the pain forced me to stop working, I was willing to try anything. I found the sheet and started sleeping grounded.

"I only wish I had done that before. I experienced a change after the very first night. I had the best night's sleep in years! The inflammation and pain eased a lot within a few days, and after four weeks the pain was gone!

"A while later, I went back to see my doctor. She was impressed with the improvement in my overall heath. She told me that the improvement showed in my face. She said that I looked like a new person. She did x-rays on my hands and could not find any inflammation. She commented that the new medications must have been really working. When I told her that I had not been taking any of the medications but just sleeping grounded, she looked puzzled. I told her I was going to keep doing it. And I have.

"Today, in 2013, I am still pain free, and in all these eight years or so I have not had to take even so much as an aspirin. I've been able to go back to work, even hold down two jobs. This thing changed my life."

AUTISM

Autism is a complex developmental disability that affects an individual's ability, in different ways and degrees, to communicate and interact with others. It typically shows up during the first three years of life and is not outgrown, causing a potentially severe emotional and financial burden on families for decades. There is no known single cause for this condition, which has risen steeply in recent years. Typical signs of autism include lack of or delay of spoken language, repetitive use of language and/or motor mannerisms (e.g., hand-flapping, twirling objects, little or no eye contact, lack of interest in peer relationships, lack of spontaneous or make-believe play, and persistent fixation on parts of objects). Sleep disturbance is often a major problem and can profoundly disrupt normal family routines.

Earthing is not a cure for autism, but over the years it's been observed to have a calming effect, improve sleep patterns, and promote better speech and socializing. Earthing reduces inflammation and strengthens the immune system and, thus, may offer additional benefit, especially in light of recent autism research revealing the presence of brain inflammation and immune system dysfunction. Earthing opens a door of hope. It may not only reduce the impact of autism on a child in a natural and simple way but also may lessen the stress level in the whole family.

Ron Petruccione, Anaheim, California, businessman: "My daughter Rosanna, now eighteen, was diagnosed with regressive moderate autism when three years old. Her condition presented itself mostly as an expressive and receptive language disorder. She often cannot produce her words fast enough and stumbles or mumbles her speech. I sometimes have to ask her, 'What did you say? Slow down!' Or in new situations and social environments where she is experiencing some anxiety, she might mix up her tenses and switch inappropriately from first to third person when speaking about herself or others.

"Rosanna has slept on a grounded sheet since early 2008. We also placed a grounded desk pad at her computer, where she spends an hour or two each day, and also have a sheet on the couch where she watches TV. So she has been getting in some extra daily grounding time.

"Within about a month after being grounded, I started to see changes. She became calmer. Her speech became more understandable. That alone has been a great improvement and stress reliever for both of us. There was less frustration showing. The anxiety wasn't there. Occasionally, I would have to tell her to slow down, but not nearly as much as before.

"She has slept better and been easier to wake up.

"Over the years in school, there has been an aide or teacher's assistant assigned to monitor her. Within a month or two after Rosanna was grounded, the aide noted in her logbook that my daughter participates more actively in the class. Lunch with the kids seemed more enjoyable for her, and the other kids seemed to be engaging her more.

"This makes me so happy. These are subtle things that can't be measured or determined by a lab test. Rosanna is now a senior in a mainstream high school! This is a big deal. She has become happier, more confident, with a little higher self-esteem. She has continued to slowly, smoothly, and

Ron Petruccione's Earthing Survey

In 2009, Ron Petruccione, the father of a teenage daughter with autism, contacted parents with autistic children around the country for the purpose of participating in an informal study involving Earthing. The idea was to provide interested parents with a grounded bed pad and have their children sleep grounded for a two-month period. The parents were asked to initially complete a twenty-question survey before the experiment and then answer the same questions on a weekly basis until the experiment ended. The questions for the survey were prepared by Mr. Petruccione, in conjunction with a Southern California mental health expert. A total of twenty-eight parents, whose children ranged in age from two to thirteen, participated in the project. The average age of the youngsters was six for girls and seven for boys. The results included the following (in percentages):

	% Before	% After
Will say good-bye		
Almost always	17.9	27.9
Almost never	46.4	23.4
Responds to familiar people		
Almost always	17.9	24.4
Almost never	32.1	15.7
Is drawn to other children		
Most of the time	17.9	33.0
Almost never	53.6	22.8
When upset, screams rather than cries tears		
Almost always	35.7	21.8
Almost never	7.1	4.1
Watches other children when they are around		
Almost always	10.7	10.2
Almost never	42.9	18.3
Actions are impulsive		
Almost always	35.7	17.8
Almost never	10.7	21.3

	% Before	% After
Has multiple allergies		
Almost always	50.0	21.8
Almost never	21.4	21.3
Likes being touched by caregivers		
Almost always	17.9	13.2
Most times	21.4	33.0
Almost never	39.3	16.2
Uses grunts or crying to communicate needs		
Almost always	17.9	18.8
Sometimes	21.4	39.1
Almost never	39.3	17.3
Sleep is calm and not restless		
Almost always	3.6	14.2
Almost never	53.6	21.8
Easygoing and flexible in schedule		
Almost always	3.6	11.7
Almost never	39.3	18.3
Easily angered		
Almost always	32.1	17.3
Almost never	7.1	16.8

surely improve, and plus over the last three years has maintained a solid 3.0 grade-point average.

"Everyone involved in this disorder knows that autism is a marathon, not a sprint. But what happened in just a couple of months and has continued is a miracle for me. Seeing things like this can make you feel like a dark cloud is lifting and can allow me to even think ahead to college. That's a possibility. I have hope to see her become a productive member of society. And that's huge, because hope is what keeps driving us parents. It takes off a little of the burden and fuels us at the same time.

"What I really like about this is that it is so very easy to use. In the the autistic community, it's often very hard to find something effective. This is not about how many supplements you can get down them or rubbing on some cream. You just put a grounded sheet on a bed, and there are real therapeutic benefits for hardly any cost in the long run. A lot of us parents are really strapped, emotionally, physically, and financially. This is something special."

Autism: Meltdowns and Moodiness Much Improved

One California mother said her five-year-old son was diagnosed with autism two years before. She described her situation thusly: "He used to wake up bright-eyed around 5:30 AM. Then he would 'burnout' from not enough sleep in the late afternoon or early evening. It was like hitting the wall. Crying. Meltdowns. Moodiness.

"We have had him sleeping grounded and he now sleeps much more soundly and for a full ten hours without waking up. He rises feeling refreshed and happy. I now realize that my son was just sleep deprived, which we all know is an issue in itself. The sheet is wonderful. He is much improved, primarily due to the sheet along with dietary and environmental changes we have made.

"Hardly anybody would know there are or have been autistic-type issues with him. The only problems are a speech delay (about one and one-half to two years behind his peers) and some residual allergies.

"In addition to sleeping grounded, our son always goes barefooted. He loves it. You should see that kid run over our landscape rocks. He has feet of steel."

BACK PAIN

Mary Mason, Haines City, Florida, retired oncology nurse: "I suffered with bad back pain for twenty-five years. It was something I had to live with because you can't take narcotic painkillers and work with patients. You have to be very clear-headed. So Tylenol was my drug of choice. That was it.

"As a nurse, I was skeptical about this Earthing idea when I first heard about it. But I decided to give it a try, and I'm sure glad I did. I've been sleeping grounded for four years and wouldn't think of sleeping any other way. Within two or three days, I noticed a difference. I remember calling my daughter at the end of the first week and telling her that my back wasn't hurting anymore.

"I don't have back pain as long as I sleep on the Earthing sheet. I use it religiously and take it with me no matter where I go. Nothing has ever worked for me like that. It has really helped my quality of life overall, and the older I get the more appreciative I am.

"From my perspective as someone who worked with ill patients for more than twenty-five years, I think that Earthing could help so many patients. You could eliminate many problems and speed the healing process. Today, they give you one pill for one thing and then another one for the side effects. And it goes on ad nauseam. Earthing could eliminate a lot of that. It could be extremely helpful in surgical recovery and chronic pain clinics."

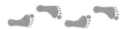

Minja Karvinen, Orimattila, Finland, counselor for the disabled: "I suffer from Modic type 1* changes, which started in 2002, and led to degeneration in six intervertebral discs, and a state of constant inflammation. Extra liquid built up in my lower back, pressing on nerves so badly that my legs didn't function. I spent six years in a wheelchair and had to take strong painkillers (up to twenty-one tablets each day). In the summer of 2009, I forced myself to get out of the wheelchair and practiced walking behind the lawnmower. The pain remained, however, and I could never be sure whether or not my legs would work. Using a back support, I was able to walk a little, but every winter the inflammation got worse and my ability to move decreased. I tried acupuncture, osteopathy, chiropractic, and nothing worked.

---

*Modic type 1 changes refer to pathological and structural degradation of vertebral bone tissue. Research suggests that this condition generates more severe pain than usual back pain in which bone tissue is normal. Three-quarters of Modic patients experience constant back pain, and nearly 70 percent are woken up by pain at night when they turn over in their sleep. MRI studies indicate that 18–58 percent of patients with lower back pain may have underlying Modic changes.

"I desired to get back into the working life and I did everything I could to not let the pain stop me. I studied for a new profession, and got a job in the field I love. The only question was, would my back last? The work is quite hard physically, sometimes I have to lift a lot of things. Every day at work I had to wear an iron back support in order to be able to do my job.

"Thanks to my employer, I learned about grounding. I obtained an Earthing mat in November 2012, which I used under my back every night. An unbelievably fast healing process began. In February 2013, new MRI pictures of my back showed all inflammation was gone! The pains disappeared and most important, I went the whole winter without using the wheelchair. I walked the whole winter! After January 2013, I didn't need the back support at work or during my free time. I was able to go to the gym, go swimming, and fishing. I still have the condition but no pain.

"In addition to my back, I also have another condition that has bothered me since I was a baby. It is called Banti's disease. When I was a child, blood didn't circulate between my liver and spleen properly and blood would come out of my mouth. Every two years, I have to have a gastroscopy to check my esophagus and stomach to see if the varices (abnormal, enlarged veins) in my esophagus show any weakening or bleeding. At the end of November 2012, I had this procedure done and the varices had disappeared. The doctor couldn't believe how it was possible, as I had had the varices for thirty-nine years. Unbelievable but true!"

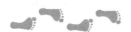

Gail LePine, South Hadley, Massachusetts, dental hygienist: "I fell off my horse many years ago and injured my coccyx. Working as a hygienist, whether I was sitting or standing, was causing a good deal of lower back pain. Just picture the position a hygienist is in for eight plus hours a day and you can well imagine the toll it takes on one's body.

"I read about Earthing in mid-2010 and started going barefoot as soon as I could. I went out in my yard, stacked wood, and did yard work. That evening, I laid down on my lawn listening to classical music for almost an hour before going to bed. I had the best night's sleep in a long time. The hip and back pain that usually would wake me up during the middle of the night was gone. I had tried chiropractic treatments and yoga. Nothing really seemed to work until I began Earthing.

"I routinely go barefoot during the warmer months and also sleep grounded. And, gratefully, as long as I continue with my Earthing routine, I am able to stay pain free. When I don't Earth regularly, the pain returns. It's an old injury and it will always haunt me."

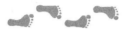

Sara Damskier, Brovst, Denmark, retired adult education director: "I suffered a back injury more than fifty years ago (diagnosed as progressive spondylolisthesis of the fifth lumbar vertebra). As I've gotten older, it has caused me increasing pain and inconvenience. Lying in bed for any length of time has been the worst of all. I have had to curl up in bed in order to press that misplaced vertebra away from the nerves that it irritates. If, for example, I would lie on my back and read in bed for just twenty minutes, it would be enormously difficult and very painful to turn over onto my side. This was also true when changing positions in the middle of the night. In both cases it would be necessary for me to lift my hips with my hands and in that manner, bit by bit, turn my body to the opposite side.

"A dramatic change occurred the very first night I slept grounded on an Earthing sheet in 2012. I was able to turn over during the night with no difficulty. The first morning I woke up lying flat on my back without pain! This was not possible before! Now I wake up in different positions, and, most important, without pain. This holds true with regard to the first movement of the morning—reaching down to put on my slippers. No pain and none of the old stiffness. It is simply fantastic!

"A year later, I continue to enjoy the relief gained from this great remedy. If I vacation away from the house where I can't get access to the Earth, the old strain and pain will start coming back. It does not, however, reappear in its most severe form right away. So it's short vacations for me and back to full protection."

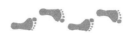

Jim Bellacera, Sacramento, California, business motivational speaker: "Ten years ago, I first heard about sleeping grounded. I thought I would be a great test case because for more than two decades I had had chronic pain from my earlier construction and cabinetmaking days. My pain problems started at around age twenty-six. I had back pain, neck pain, and carpal tunnel pain. During one job, I jumped off a trailer while carrying a cabinet, and I crushed my back. That act alone caused endless pain.

"Nothing I ever did ever seemed to help, from seeing doctors and getting regular back treatments to taking 800 milligrams of ibuprofen two or three times a day and sometimes other anti-inflammatories as well.

"And, son of a gun, I woke up in disbelief the morning after the first night I slept grounded. 'No, this can't be,' I said. 'My back doesn't hurt.'

"Not only didn't it hurt, but after a day or two, I didn't have to reach for my daily dose of ibuprofen horse pills.

"Getting up in the mornings had been a challenge. I would roll out of bed, use my arms, and do kind of a push-up with my feet touching the ground so I could stand straight up without bending my back. That changed right away with Earthing. I was able to get out of bed with no pain. Today, I don't have pain in the back, neck, or wrists. It's been an absolute blessing."

INFLAMMATION OF THE BLOOD VESSELS

Behcet's syndrome causes problems in many parts of the body, including skin sores, swelling of parts of the eyes, pain, swelling and stiffness of joints, meningitis, blood clots, inflammation of the digestive system, and blindness. The condition mostly affects people in their twenties and thirties. There is no cure. Treatment focuses on reducing pain and preventing serious problems.

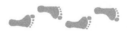

Randy Gillett, Upland, California, retired manager of a bedding manufacturing company: "In 1999, I was diagnosed with Behcet's syndrome. I was left profoundly deaf and in a constant state of vertigo, a result of lack of blood flow to my inner ears and vestibular (balance) centers caused by inflammation.

"I also lost sight in one eye and had constant joint pain, especially in my blistered and swollen feet. I developed ulcers in my mouth and lesions on various parts of my body, and I was left extremely fatigued.

"After months of medications and bed rest, I was able to return to work but still had to take multiple medications to reduce inflammation and regulate my immune system.

"At the end of each work week, I would be very fatigued and spent most of my weekends sleeping. My feet got progressively worse with pain and swelling. I had to start wearing sandals to work and kept a pair of house slippers by my desk to wear around the office. My doctor prescribed Vioxx for the pain and inflammation in my feet. I fully expected that some day I would not be able to walk, and chronic pain was something I must live with. Between the medications and pain, I would be up three to six times a night and sometimes couldn't sleep at all.

"I started sleeping grounded in 2004. After the third night, my feet were no longer swollen. I was able to wiggle my toes and didn't have any pain. It was unbelievable. Every morning after that was like waking up with new feet. I was able to stop taking the prednisone, the Vioxx, and a blood-thinning medication. I was sleeping deeper than ever and most of the time completely through the night. On weekends, I was now able to enjoy my leisure time.

"Ear cochlear implant surgery, along with behind-the-ear sound enhancement technology, has helped my hearing on one side, although it is nowhere near what God gave me. I do not expect the grounding to restore my hearing and cure the vertigo or completely restore the damage done to my body, but I wake up pain free every morning.

"I sleep grounded every night and will always do so. It keeps the inflammation in check and helps me to be as healthy as possible. Because of grounding I am able to function pretty good. It has kept me from having major flare-ups for all these years.

"I still see my doctor every four months and get blood work done every year. My doctor tells me my blood tests are like that of a man in his thirties, twenty to thirty years younger than my actual age.

"I tried working for five years after getting better, but everyday business was just too stressful. The amount of energy and focus to try and stay balanced and understand what was being said was exhausting, and driving was dangerous. So I keep busy around the house, watching aging parents, and doing things to help wherever I can with family and friends. If I am busy doing yard work and chores around the house, the pain in my feet sometimes creeps back, and by the end of the day I am ready for sleep and grounding, but again in the morning I feel good and pain free.

"I can't express enough how much grounding has made my life better. I feel blessed, and I am happy to be alive."

JET LAG

Jim Bagnola, Austin, Texas, leadership consultant and author of *Becoming a Professional Human Being.* "In my work, I travel all over the world, so jet lag is always an issue. In my experience, going barefoot and sleeping grounded are the fastest ways to realign to a far-flung time zone. I also sleep more soundly, with more lucid dreaming, and feel stronger physically.

"In the past I have tried all kinds of treatments, remedies, and gadgets to counteract jet lag. Walking on grass and sleeping grounded works for me the most effectively. After returning home to Texas from a recent trip to France, England, and Romania, I recovered within a couple of days. It would otherwise take me a week after an extended trip like that.

"When I arrive at foreign destinations and check into my hotel, I walk barefoot on grass wherever I can find it. This has been a hilarious experience at times. I travel to Romania quite a bit, and in downtown Bucharest I take advantage of a good patch of grass in front of the National Theatre, next door to the Intercontinental Hotel. As I do my twenty minutes of barefoot walking there, people will often stop and watch me circling the grassy area in my bare feet. Some ask what I am doing. I attempt to tell them about grounding and jet lag, and they look at me as if I am crazy. Many cannot speak English so it makes the situation rather humorous. I did get a bee sting once so I have to be careful where I walk. But otherwise it works great."

LUPUS

Autoimmune disorders are unpredictable. Flare-ups and return of symptoms can occur because of various types of stress, including emotional stress, seasonal allergies, and overwork. In such situations, individuals who have been routinely sleeping grounded often benefit by maximizing their hours of grounding.

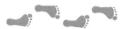

Katie McGuinness, Santa Inez Valley, California, former corporate general counsel: "Lupus is 'the great imitator,' a disease that hides behind a smokescreen of possible diagnoses and often leads to frustration over doctors' inability to diagnose what's wrong.

"Diagnosis revolves around eleven criteria based on physical symptoms and blood tests. If you have four of them, you are considered to have the disease. The bottom line is that lupus is an inflammatory process affecting joints and internal organs. I have had both shoulders, elbows, wrists, and knees involved, and such pain that I took aspirin by the handful as well as other painkillers. I learned that you don't get rid of the pain but you do get erosive gastritis and damage the digestive tract.

"Lupus first manifested in 1999 with kidney dysfunction. Suddenly, I was producing very little urine and put on fourteen pounds in five days. My blood pressure spiked. I had waste products in my blood and urine. A doctor said I had idiopathic glomerulonephritis, but I wasn't such an idiot that I swallowed that diagnosis. Idiopathic is doc speak for 'we don't know the cause.' With diuretics, the fluid came off and my lab results eventually went back to normal.

"Similar, but less severe, episodes occurred over the next four years. I had frequent joint pain and fatigue. My hands and feet became swollen and red at times, a sign of inflammatory arthritis. Symptoms worsened. I was prescribed an antimalarial drug, a first-line, anti-inflammatory medication used against lupus. This approach worked for about eighteen months and kept the symptoms under control.

"Lupus has different triggers. I learned, for instance, that sun exposure could trigger a flare-up. I was living in Southern California and getting a lot of sun. That was my catalyst for starting down a pharmaceutical road to steroids. Fatigue turned to exhaustion. At times I was short of breath and even conversation could be a challenge.

"Finally, lab tests revealed one of the lupus hallmarks: antinuclear antibodies. My body was creating antibodies to fight the nuclei of its own cells. I had become autoimmune. Initially, I got by with a three-week course of steroids that lowered the pain back to tolerable. I regained strength. But then the flare-ups became harder to control. The steroid dosage went up and there was growing concern about potential side effects, such as osteoporosis.

"In 2009, the steroids were having less and less effect, and the fatigue was debilitating. Even sleeping ten hours a day didn't produce enough energy to let me do the things I liked to do. I couldn't cook or walk the dogs. Along with this came mental fog.

"At this point, my rheumatologist prescribed CellCept, an immune-suppressant drug used when steroids aren't helping. It reduces inflammation and autoantibody production in patients with autoimmune disorders. This, and other similar drugs, are used also after organ transplants to prevent immune-system rejection. The medications, however, can weaken your defenses and render you more vulnerable to cancer and other very nasty things. Side effects include high blood pressure, kidney and liver problems, and susceptibility to infection. These are not drugs you take lightly. I told my doctor I would consider this option carefully. I was confused about what to do.

"Luckily, nature intervened. A friend told me about Earthing. I was willing to try most anything, so I started sleeping grounded. To my great surprise, I started feeling better, had more energy, and my thinking became clearer. Several weeks later, I had my regular appointment with the rheumatologist. I told him, 'It's really strange but I'm starting to feel like my old self again.' He told me this was the first time in the five years he knew me that my bloodwork was normal. None of the hallmark factors for lupus were present, including the antinuclear antibody results that had been positive for ten years!

"Six months after I started grounding, I was taking my good health and energy for granted. I was walking my dogs twice a day, taking tai chi classes, studying photography, and participating in two weekly strength-training classes to prevent osteoporosis. Unfortunately, the years of steroids had seriously weakened my bones. But every night I was sleeping grounded and only wishing I had started sooner.

"In April 2011, my blood levels still showed no antinuclear antibodies or other markers of inflammation! A few weeks later, however, I felt returning symptoms, including achy joints and knuckles, and inflamed blood vessels. I was sleeping grounded routinely, so I started Earthing as much as possible during the day. I used a mat under my forearms that grounded me during hours of writing and then used a grounded wristband while reading or watching television. I was grounded almost 24/7.

"Within days I was feeling better and with less pain. After three weeks, I was much, much better. My energy and vitality levels returned to even above what they were before my 'wobble/relapse.' An elevated red rash from inflamed blood vessels had also disappeared.

"A mutual friend perhaps put it best when he said: 'Katie is doing so well she is shell-shocked with wellness!' I had also lost twenty-five pounds in a year. My long-term dosage of steroids had caused weight gain and that situation gradually reversed itself after I discontinued the drugs.

"When routine blood and urine tests in early 2013 suggested my lupus might be staging a comeback, I was puzzled. I checked my Earthing connections and found that the ground rod I was using had somehow disappeared over the winter. I fixed that fast. After eight weeks of intense 24/7 grounding, my lab results returned to normal. My energy has remained robust ever since, and I have added square dancing to my slate of activities.

"I will be forever grateful to Earthing for restoring my health and vitality. I don't consider myself to be cured. But I do consider myself to be in remission. I've been given a second chance at life."

LYME DISEASE AND EARTHING—GO SLOW

Lyme disease is a bacterial infection transmitted by the bite of an infected tick. The condition was first reported in the United States in 1975 and has now been documented in many other parts of the world. The Centers for Disease Control and Prevention announced in 2013 that some 300,000 Americans are diagnosed annually. Lyme disease is usually treatable soon after an infectious bite with at least a month of antibiotics. However, it can become chronic when undertreated or untreated. Early symptoms can include a bull's eye rash, flu-like symptoms, and joint pain. Later symptoms can become disabling and include neurological manifestations like facial palsy, loss of cognitive abilities, sleep disturbances, and heart abnormalities.

Alix Mayer is the co-founder of www.spirochicks.com, a collaborative Lyme lifestyle blog: "Earthing is profoundly healing for Lyme, as I and many others have discovered. I first grounded myself in 2010, while attending an out-of-town health conference. I felt a sense of calm immediately after placing an Earthing band around the ball of my foot. I fell asleep faster and slept a bit better than normal for someone with normally raging insomnia. Imagine doing that in a hotel room! Moreover, my permanent headache—a problem for sixteen years—abated significantly at the conference.

"When I returned home, I continued using the band. My sleep improved, and after a few weeks I felt brave enough to stop cold turkey my prescription sleep medication. I had no trouble sleeping through the night and for sure didn't miss the medication or the awful 'hangovers' it gave me. I'm not recommending this to anyone on sleep meds, just telling my experience. I also dumped sleep supplements except melatonin because my body makes less than normal melatonin.

"I began sleeping like a baby with deliciously long nights, sometimes for twelve hours. How welcome this was after many episodes of all-night insomnia during the previous eight years.

"I then decided to get a recovery bag, one of the grounded sheets, thinking that 'more is better.' It turned out to be too much exposure in my case. The first night, I couldn't get to sleep. The next day I had my trademark post-insomnia symptoms that render me nonfunctional: dizziness, a feeling of being 'drunk,' and terrible pain in my head and body. My guess was that Earthing had caused a setback of insomnia due to amplified Herxheimer and/or detoxification reactions.

"Individuals undergoing Lyme treatment sometimes experience Herxheimer reactions, an odd phenomenon where one feels worse because bacterial die-off produces an inflammatory event. Some people associate fatigue, nausea, and fever with 'herxing.' Such reactions can also cause previous symptoms to temporarily reappear.

"Earthing may also increase the body's ability to detoxify—the actual cleaning out through our organs of dead bacterial debris, such as Lyme spirochetes, and their resultant endotoxins. We can have detoxification reactions when the liver, kidneys, lymphatics, colon, or skin become over-loaded and unable to manage the demands placed on them. Long-term Lyme patients have notoriously impaired detoxification. It's possible that Earthing increases the capacity of one or more of these systems to elim-inate toxins, but the body may retain bottlenecks in other organs that then get overloaded. There are many detox symptoms, including fatigue, joint or muscle pain, skin rashes, sleep disturbances, irritability, and headaches.

"Despite my setback, I still strongly believed that Earthing was good for me, so I decided to use the band again around my foot, which had generated wonderful benefits without discomfort. I took the recovery bag off my bed for a while. The strategy worked. I did pretty well with sleep and was gradually able to build back up to Earthing my entire body with the sheet, without an uptick in insomnia.

"Undoubtedly, my reaction was a Lyme-specific reaction: too much Earth-ing, too quickly. This experience is actually quite common among Lyme patients. It doesn't mean that Earthing's benefits—like pain reduction and better sleep—will not occur. It just means we need to go slower with Earthing. Gradually build up the duration and amount of the body that is Earthed, so we don't get slammed with a Herxheimer or detox reaction.

"Lee Cowden, M.D., a well-known integrative physician and natural Lyme practitioner, directs Lyme patients to start Earthing for fifteen to thirty minutes a day, building up to three hours while awake. Once you can Earth for three hours in the day, he says you can then try sleeping grounded overnight.

"Due to oftentimes quick provocation of reactions, some of my friends with Lyme have started very, very slowly, only touching the metallic con-tact on a grounded band for five or ten minutes per day. Some got a reac-tion, sometimes described as nausea, sometimes described as 'detoxing too quickly,' even at this very minimal level. Some, like me, reacted quite pos-itively at first. Many reported that once they weathered the temporary roughness, they experienced less pain and fewer headaches, better sleep, clearer thinking, a more alkaline body, and even improved excretion of heavy metals. Others never endured a negative reaction at all and enjoyed the benefits. Still others report no apparent symptom benefits. We don't know yet how many Lyme patients fall in each group.

"Because grounding causes Herxheimer and detox reactions in Lyme patients, it must be inherently healing. It's hard to imagine that touching Mother Earth could cause ill health. What fascinates me, and demands study, are the reasons why the Earth may help Lyme patients heal.

"Some possibilities include the ability to thin the blood, which may allow the antibiotics used to treat Lyme to penetrate more deeply into tissue and access spirochetes. Thinner blood may also contribute to better detox function. Increased blood oxygenation from Earthing might be detrimental to circulating spirochetes, causing more die-off than normal. Earthing may also disrupt spirochetes from forming cysts, a theoretical Lyme-defense mechanism.

"Even without Lyme-specific research, we can begin to create an Earthing strategy. My personal strategy is to sleep and work at my desk grounded. I also try to walk barefoot on the beach and wear conductive flip-flops outside.

"I'm happy that after more than three years of herbal Lyme treatment and after a sharp and unmistakable reduction of symptoms starting with daily Earthing in 2010, I was able to stop treating my Lyme in spring 2012! I've had a substantial recovery. Severe headaches and brain fog are largely a thing of the past. My joint pain is much reduced. I feel calmer and ready to sleep as soon as I connect to the Earth for the night. Sleep is still a demon I fight each night, but it is more good than bad, and my baseline is much improved."

MEN'S HEALTH

Psychotherapist Jed Diamond, Ph.D., a well-known author of books on men's health (including *Stress Relief for Men*), regards Earthing as "probably the simplest energy-healing tool anyone can use. Getting in touch with the Earth is more than a metaphor, it is a physiological reality."

He shared this story with us: "After I finished my last book, I told my son I needed a physical challenge to ground me after spending so much time 'in my head.' I wasn't quite prepared for his suggestion. 'Let's train and run a marathon,' he enthusiastically told me. I'm sixty-six-years-old and hadn't run more than a 10K (half marathon) in my entire life. But I agreed to give it a try. 'Hey, we'll pick a race where there's a 10K and a marathon,' he told me. 'I'll run the marathon, you can run the 10K if you want.'

"But things didn't work out as planned. I had read the Earthing book and began using what I'd learned. He thought Earthing sounded 'weird' and didn't want to try it. Halfway through our six-month training program he dropped out due to injuries. I completed the training and ran my first marathon ever. I continued to use Earthing on a daily basis hoping it would help me stay healthy and stress-free. It sure looks like it did.

"As a healthcare provider, I'm always looking for ways to improve the health of my clients. I have found that the benefits of Earthing go way beyond helping people who want to improve their sports performance. I specialize in men's health and have 'prescribed' Earthing to many clients for dealing with common low energy and chronic pain. As an example, a fifty-four-year-old client who had suffered from severe neck and back pain for many years found that Earthing was remarkably effective. He was quite amazed that connecting to the Earth could relieve his pain and allow him to sleep peacefully for the first time in a long time.

"Another client who was taking multiple medications to deal with low energy and chronic fatigue found that Earthing recharged his battery. 'I have a lot more energy with which to enjoy my life,' he said. 'I no longer nod off after dinner or have to limit my activities. I sleep better and I feel better. And, best of all, I no longer have to use the medications that I thought I'd have to take the rest of my life.'

"These are typical things I hear from clients."

Less Nighttime Urination

Many men, middle aged and up, have reported less urgency to get up at night to urinate, a result we believe from reduced inflammation of the prostate gland.

Here are several typical comments:

- **From a fifty-nine-year-old male after sleeping grounded for eight months:** "The main reason for trying Earthing was to improve inflammation and soreness in my left foot. That problem went away within the month. I can also say that I need to use the washroom much less during the night—used to be two to three times per night, and now only once if at all."

- **"From a sixty-three-year-old male, sleeping grounded for more than two years:** "I only pee once a night and sometimes not at all. Before Earthing, I might urinate three or four times. Doc says my prostate is normal for my age with some enlargement."

SLEEP APNEA

An estimated 2 to 7 percent of adults worldwide have sleep apnea. This means episodes of impaired breathing and disturbed sleep caused by a narrowing of soft tissue in the upper airway. Apnea reduces oxygen in the blood and prompts arousal from sleep. A continuous positive airway pressure (CPAP) machine is widely used as a remedy. It delivers a stream of compressed air via a hose to a nasal pillow, nose mask, or full-face mask. The pressure keeps the airway open. Researchers think that obstructive sleep apnea activates an inflammatory response in the body that may contribute to cardiovascular disease.

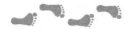

Beverley Shoemaker, Parry Sound, Ontario, Canada, retired critical care nurse: "I am an insomniac with sleep apnea! I began using a CPAP sleep regimen prior to sleeping grounded. I improved somewhat on the CPAP, but I hit the jackpot when I began using Earthing.

"I go to a deeper level of sleep, with much more REM sleep, and with fewer awakenings. Consequently, I have more reserve to get through the day. Even if my night is shorter for other reasons, I have plenty of daytime energy. This is hugely important for me.

"I never, ever want to sleep without Earthing again. I feel many on CPAP would benefit by combining it with Earthing. I think they would be much less aware of their respiratory apparatus if they were sleeping 'deeper' with grounding.

"This is a huge quality-of-life difference for me."

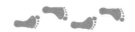

Daryl James, Palm Springs, California, business consultant: "Increasingly, over a period of a few years, I would wake up a few times a night gasping for breath. Finally, I went to a sleep clinic. The tests indicated that I had a moderate case of sleep apnea, with episodes where I would stop breathing for twenty seconds at a time. A lot of sleep apnea patients die in their sleep. I didn't want to be one of them.

"I was told to get a CPAP machine. I did just that. I used it every night and it helped me sleep without interruption, but I didn't like using the device. It's not very comfortable.

"After hearing about grounding and how it improved sleep, I decided to give it a try and see if it could possibly help my situation. It did!

"There were times when the CPAP face mask was too uncomfortable so I removed it. And even without it, I was able to get through the night without any problem for quite a while. I noticed this within a few months of grounding. Over time, however, my apnea has worsened and I have had to use the CPAP routinely, but my Earthing sheets remain an integral tool with which to combat the problem.

"I have found also that I have more energy during the day. That means a lot to somebody in his eighties.

"In addition, my blood pressure stabilized since being grounded. Previously, my blood pressure control wasn't as good as my doctor would have liked it to be even though I was taking medication.

STRESS RELIEF

Surveys indicate that adults regard themselves under much more stress than ever. In the United States, an estimated 75 to 90 percent of visits to primary care physicians are for stress-related problems. Yet, most people don't realize the degree of damage that stress inflicts on their personal health. "I'm just a little stressed," they'll say, as if chronic stress equates to caffeinated edginess. Stress equates with strain on the body, and too much of it brings trouble in many forms. Stress can lead to high blood pressure, heart attacks, stroke, sudden death, depression, insomnia, headaches, muscle spasms, memory loss, weight gain, abdominal fat, erectile dysfunction, and lack of libido. It undermines the body's defenses and thus increases the risk, frequency, and severity of colds, allergic reactions, and autoimmune disorders. In brief, stress can kill your heart, shrink your brain, destroy your resistance to illness, and shorten your life.

Stress impacts your adrenal glands directly. They are the organs that produce stress hormones that react to acute stress (adrenaline and the "fight-or-flight" reaction) and chronic stress (cortisol). In this process, cortisol becomes elevated and depleted, interfering with sleep and blood glucose control, fueling anxiety and depression, and depleting the immune system. New research shows that chronic psychological stress and abnormal levels of cortisol impair the body's ability to control inflammation, a breakdown that adds to understanding the role of stress in multiple disorders.

Earthing has a beneficial effect on cortisol and other hormones; it calms the nervous system and reduces inflammation and thus offers an effective and natural remedy for counteracting stress and adrenal exhaustion. We strongly believe that one of the major stresses on the body is something that few people realize: the lack of connection with the Earth.

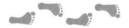

Ashley Kane, Decatur, Georgia, disabled former attorney: "Over the past ten years, I have transformed from a healthy, thirty-year-old attorney to a forty-something on disability. All of my illnesses have involved inflammation and the adrenal glands.

"In 2002, I was a new attorney, loving the fast pace. The stress was like a drug to me. That year, I developed Sjögren's syndome, an autoimmune disease. My immune system was attacking my body and creating inflammation. The next year, I developed chronic hives, a further result of inflammation in my body.

"In 2005, I developed whooping cough and was ill for six weeks. The following year I developed an extremely rare flesh-eating pneumonia. I became septic and was in a narcotically induced coma for two weeks with encephalitis and acute respiratory distress syndrome. My adrenal glands failed due to the stress put on my immune system. The doctors told my husband that I would likely be a vegetable if I ever awoke. Miraculously, I woke up with my mental faculties intact. I returned to full-time work after eight weeks, in denial about the severity of my condition.

"Within weeks, I developed chronic fatigue immune dysfunction syndrome (CFIDS). My adrenals were exhausted. I couldn't sleep, even with sleeping pills. I couldn't eat. I felt constantly wired due to a resurgence of Epstein-Barr virus. My anxiety went through the roof. I began getting recurrent pneumonia due to lung damage and lack of immunity. Because I was bedridden, I had to go on disability.

"In 2010, an experimental antiviral drug improved my CFIDS so that I was no longer bedridden. However, in 2012, I developed dysautonomia, a malfunction of the autonomic nervous system. I became very sensitive to exercise, sometimes throwing up after exerting myself. I became dizzy if I didn't drink water and take salt at timed intervals throughout the day. I had to sleep sitting up because of bad bed spins. I had adrenaline surges and low blood sugar where I would almost faint. I often could not get up in the morning and slept until noon. I had no energy and felt depressed. It's hard not to be a miserable person when you are miserable.

"I began trying every treatment I could find. I did graded exercise, acupuncture, Chinese herbs, diet, and nutraceuticals. I got all sorts of blood tests, nutrition evaluations, and food allergy testing. Nothing worked. After a year, I gave up on ever improving the dysautonomia. I had become so obsessed with feeling better that my stress levels were at an all-time high.

"Around this time, I started getting neck pain that wouldn't go away. Having to sleep sitting up compounded the problem. It was debilitating, so I started researching pain relief. That's when I stumbled upon Earthing.

"I started sleeping grounded. My husband thought I was daffy and refused to sleep on the Earthing sheet. On the first night, I had an intense die-off reaction, something that happens to people with CFIDS who have chronic viral infections, when their immune system or a drug they are taking starts destroying the pathogens. The die-off made it difficult to sleep.

"I had never experienced die-off before from anything but potent antiviral drugs, so I did some online research. I found reports from people with Lyme disease and CFIDS who developed die-off symptoms when Earthing. The die-off may be due to the thinning of the blood that occurs with grounding, better allowing the immune system to attack and destroy pathogens.

"On the fourth evening, we went on a church retreat in the wilderness. Once there, I realized I had forgotten my salt. Panic!! My husband scoured the campgrounds trying unsuccessfully to find extra salt. I finally decided to tough it out. That night, I had no dizziness, no nausea, and I slept like a rock. I was shocked.

"Once we got home, I decided to test whether I still needed salt and water for my dysautonomia. I purposely got extremely dehydrated and had no salt, and I felt fine all day and slept well that night. The next day, I felt the same, and it's been the same every day since. I no longer have nausea. I never get dizzy unless I go a full twelve hours without drinking. My dysautonomia is much improved, and I believe that it will continue to get better.

"After a short period of time Earthing, I noticed numerous other changes, as well:

"1) My adrenal fatigue seemed to disappear. Even though I hadn't slept well those first nights due to die-off, I woke up with more energy than when I was sleeping twelve hours before. I no longer needed to sleep until noon. I actually felt like I had before I suffered from adrenal failure in 2006.

"2) My anxiety and anger lifted. My husband noticed a rapid change in my moods and my energy. After seeing such positive changes in me, he decided to sleep grounded as well. He was glad that he did. He experienced significant relief from a painful shoulder condition.

"3) My neck pain disappeared after three weeks.

"4) For my entire adult life I have had extremely painful periods due to cramping and horrible PMS. I have had to take numerous painkillers every month to combat the pain. It was so bad on several occasions that I had to go to the emergency room. Now, my PMS and cramps have seemingly disappeared. My husband used to steer a wide path around me during that time of month because of my mood swings and unpleasantness. He is pleasantly surprised by the change.

"Sleeping grounded has greatly reduced the inflammation and taken care of the stress by restoring balance and rhythm to my adrenals. I feel lighter, happier, more peaceful, less stressed. I have finally found a major healing tool, one that my body has been missing my entire life, and I am so grateful. I will never sleep ungrounded again!"

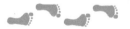

Scott Hyatt, Northern California law enforcement officer: "I work in narcotics, and my life can be very stressful from just the people I come in contact with, to making time for court, and for family and everything else. In my work, I can be one minute on surveillance, sitting there and nothing's happening. And the next minute, I'm out of the car and running, trying to get my raid vest on and my weapon out. So the stresses are from zero up to 100 miles an hour at any given time.

"Sleep takes a hit in all this irregularity. My sleep routine was skewed at best. So there's a lot of fatigue. In my job I've broken my foot, my hand, my nose, and my wrist. So there are also aches and pains from that, as well as a stiff back from wearing gun belts and raid vests.

"I've been sleeping grounded for about six years. And it made a huge difference. I used to be up a lot in the middle of the night—tossing and turning, fluffing my pillow, getting up, stretching, getting back into bed. And after I started using the bed pad, I've been getting a better quality of sleep—maybe not as much time as I would like because we still have strange hours we have to work with, but the quality of sleep really improved.

"There's also been a big difference in the aches and pains. They're gone. I didn't even really notice it until after six months or so. I woke up one morning and got right out of bed and there were no aches and pains, no sore back, no sore feet. It was amazing. I had probably not had any pain or stiffness before that but hadn't noticed it.

"I'm an avid runner, and so I'm used to the aches and pains of my ankles, knees, and hip flexors. They were gone as well. When I was out running later that day, it just kept reoccurring to me that something had changed and it wasn't my job, it wasn't my eating habits, it wasn't anything else. I could only put it to the bed pad.

"When I would run races—like five kilometers—and trying to beat my friends I would be running faster than when I'm out just on my own. The next morning I would usually be plenty sore and achy. The bed pad has taken that away as well. The aches are minimal. It's amazing."

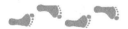

Brad Graham, Lakewood, California, firefighter: "This job, as you can imagine, involves a lot of stress, physically and mentally. You never know what you are going to face at any particular time of the day or night.

"You could be asleep at 1:00 AM, and you get a call. It may be to respond to a fire or to a situation where people are trapped in a car that's been in an accident. You go from deep rest to fast and furious action and saving lives.

"When you get back to the station, it's hard to get the scenes of what you have been through out of your mind. If you rescue somebody who was injured, you wonder if they will be okay. And you may think about what you could have done different to affect the outcome.

"Because of the nature of the work, sometimes it is very, very difficult to get back to sleep after a call. Sometimes I'll lie in bed for hours. Sometimes I'll even get up, take a shower, and go to the kitchen and read the paper.

"When I sleep grounded, I find I am able to go back to sleep after a call in what I would consider a decent time period. Maybe twenty minutes versus two and a half hours. I also notice that I sleep deeper and feel more rested when I get up in the morning. I'm more rested, but still alert.

"There seems to be a physical benefit as well. Our type of work can be quite strenuous. I think some of the issues that firefighters face, especially as the years take their toll on us, is that our knees get a little stiff. Or, as we get older, we develop back problems. Ever since I've been sleeping grounded, my knees don't feel as stiff as they used to. I like to maintain my strength by lifting weights. For quite a while, I pretty much wasn't able to do squats. Now, at the gym, I can perform squats again. And I'm able to run better than before."

STRESS AND ELECTROSENSITIVITY

Over the years, people have told us they are "electrosensitive" and suffer from exposure to common electromagnetic fields, such as from household wiring, cordless phones, cellphones, and Wi-Fi. Research in Europe suggests that 3 to 6 percent of the population may be affected. We believe that such individuals frequently have a background of chronic stress and, as a result, weakened adrenal glands. Some have told us, in fact, that they have been diagnosed with adrenal problems. Typically, adrenal weakness goes undiagnosed and symptoms of stress are usually treated with antianxiety drugs, antidepressants, and sleeping pills. As described earlier in this section, weakened adrenals can lead to a host of problems. Electrosensitivity may be one of them. Doctors familiar with adrenal exhaustion indicate that individuals with this problem commonly have allergies, chronic pain and fatigue, and sensitivity to multiple environmental factors, such as wind, heat, noise, cold, certain foods, and chemicals. Earthing helps people cope better with these problems.

Step Sinatra, whose electrosensitivity story you will read next, is the eldest son of coauthor Stephen Sinatra. Despite all the best care that Dr. Sinatra could arrange, he and his family watched anxiously while Step's health deteriorated over several years. "There was great fear we might lose Step," according to Dr. Sinatra. "He has made a remarkable recovery, literally from death's door."

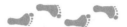

Step Sinatra, Calistoga, California, entrepreneur: "In the late 1990s, I was trading stocks on Wall Street, on a floor with a hundred guys surrounded by a battery of computers, phones, and electronics. I worked in this intense environment nonstop throughout the day. I used two cell phones and my monthly bills were $5,000.

"I was in constant overdrive, filled with a zest for life and a desire to experience it all. I was young, strong, and healthy. I worked hard, took enormous risks, and felt I could handle it all. I was living a high-intensity New York City lifestyle. I had an apartment on the forty-third floor that faced the World Trade Towers and a battery of electromagnetic antennas eight blocks away.

"For four years I didn't sleep much. I was stressed. In time, I began to feel something affecting my health. I thought it was the intensity of my work. Then things started to go wrong. I developed ear, eye, and nose problems, a chronic cough, and major congestion. My symptoms got worse, but I didn't stop and listen. I felt I would get healthy later. I was making serious money and living what I thought was a successful lifestyle.

"However, at one point, I had chest pains that my father thought might be coronary artery spasms or an early warning of a heart attack. I was twenty-five years old!

"The experience stopped me in my tracks. I realized I was really beaten down and was smart enough to know when to throw in the towel. In 2001, after the attack on the World Trade Towers, I moved to Colorado and worked on getting my health back. But I just kept deteriorating with weakness and weight loss. It was scary.

"I set up a small office in Boulder—a trading operation—and filled it with wireless networks and cordless phones, not knowing the harm they were causing me. I worked and slept there, so I was getting hit with electromagnetic fields (EMFs) day and night. I still didn't understand what I had. All I knew was I was getting worse, with weight loss, weakness, severe bloating and gas, inability to digest certain foods, muscle pains, injuries, sleep issues, and food allergies.

"I consulted with nutritionists, acupuncturists, alternative therapists, and conventional doctor after doctor. My father was also trying to help me. I did blood test after inconclusive blood test. Nobody knew what was wrong. I kept fading away, losing two or three pounds a month no matter what I did.

"I had to get out of trading, but I still needed my laptop and cell phone because I worked for myself. I began to strongly suspect that EMFs were harmful because exposure to them made me feel worse. I don't know if I was always sensitive to EMFs or developed an extreme sensitivity on Wall Street from all the stress.

"My father had me see some of the best doctors in the country he knew. Nobody could figure it out. One time I spent $20,000 at a famous clinic and they couldn't figure anything out. They just said I had endocrine problems. It was scary knowing that something was seriously wrong and yet no doctor knew why I got sick or why I was doing so poorly. All I knew was that I had become defenseless and vulnerable.

"I reached a culmination point in 2007 when I developed a parasite infection. I lost another thirty-five pounds within several weeks. My body completely shut down, and I had to be hospitalized. I was six feet tall and weighed eighty-three pounds. My liver, kidney, and blood tests were off the charts! I had to be fed via intravenous nutrition. That's what saved me, along with the prayers and love from family and friends.

"The doctors gave me a 1 percent chance. If I did live, they had no idea what my life would be like because my body had eaten most of itself. I was in excruciating pain. I couldn't go to the bathroom because I was pretty much paralyzed. There were times I was so weak that if a visitor walked into the room talking on a cell phone I would feel nauseous. If somebody brought a laptop to show me pictures, I couldn't look at it for more than a minute. I was that sensitive and had become increasingly aware of my sensitivity.

"One night I almost choked while taking a sip of water, and I thought I was gone. So did my dad, who was with me. But in that moment something Divine manifested, a sort of spiritual awakening or angelic intervention. I suddenly knew that we create our fears, dreams, and almost everything else. It was the worst and best moment of my life at the same time. I realized that with the intention of spirit I could create anything. I asked God for a miracle, and my prayer was answered. I felt reconnected and knew I would recover.

"I started to reverse course and improve. After forty days, I was finally strong enough to leave the hospital. I was still super fragile, though. My father talked to me around this time about Earthing, even just sitting with my bare feet on the grass. As the weather warmed up, I started sitting, standing, and walking barefoot a bit. I noticed my strength coming back slowly. I made sure that there were very few electromagnetic gadgets in my vicinity.

"I became extremely wary about my environment and cleared out any electrical and electronic stuff. I felt and slept better. I didn't use a computer for the first nine months out of the hospital. I wouldn't even look at one. I stopped speaking on a cell phone unless absolutely necessary and that might be only once or twice a month. I only used a corded phone and a computer connected to a landline. No wireless.

"Shortly after I got out of the hospital, I started sleeping grounded. It was amazing. The first few nights, I got perhaps six or seven hours of sleep, but I woke up feeling better each day—compared to sleeping nine or ten hours previously and waking up feeling poorly. I felt such a dramatic boost in energy and health that I have not slept ungrounded since.

"I've actually been able to handle more EMFs as I got stronger. When I use a computer, I have my feet on a grounded floor mat, so I'm able to stay on the computer much longer than before. If I'm not grounded, after about ten minutes I get hot, sweaty, and uncomfortable. When I travel, I take my grounding sheet with me. I take off my shoes and ground myself during the day whenever and wherever I can.

"Today, at 150 pounds, I am stronger than I have been in years. I'm blessed to be alive."

YOGA TEACHER, MOTHER, AND STUDENTS— ALL FEELING THE DIFFERENCE

Louise Horgan, Dublin, Ireland, yoga teacher: "I have been Earthing for two years and am continually astonished at the overhaul this has created in my body, mind, and, dare I say, spirit.

"I have psoriasis (the Irish are plagued with skin disorders!) and have seen marked improvement, especially in the summer months when I combine sleeping grounded with a lot of barefoot time, and, of course, the sun helps, too. I have plaques on both elbows and knees and they have diminished significantly in size and redness.

"My experience has inspired me to spread the word, and those who have gotten grounded have reported wonderful benefits ranging from hyper children becoming calmer to a rapid healing of a chronic, painful foot ulcer resistant to medication.

"My mother, chronically ill for two years with transverse myelitis, an inflammatory neurological disorder of the spinal cord, was massively helped after just three nights of sleeping grounded. The pain in her legs diminished significantly; however, it was the sense of well-being she felt from Earthing that changed her perspective on her illness and within those days she began her recovery, which now, two years later, is complete.

"As a yoga teacher, I now take my classes outdoors during the summer to a Victorian square next to the studio. My students always comment on their experience practicing on the grass (usually a bit damp from morning dew) as being exceptionally healing."

HAPPINESS

Tino Phuthego, Gaborone, Botswana, government pilot: "I have studied alternative health extensively to help my family and friends enjoy a better level of health. I've had pretty good results although we were still niggled by this or that. Then I discovered Earthing in 2011 and I have to say it is one of the most powerful things anybody can do for their health.

"Our sleep is better and we are all more energetic. My wife is a dentist and in the past was usually exhausted after a day at work. It's obvious now that she has more energy after work.

"We still cough and have a cold now and then, but it's getting less and less. We have changed significantly in a very subtle way.

"The biggest blessing, and maybe the most subtle, has been happiness. I notice we have become happier, like when we were younger. Even our kids (ages three and eight) have become bubbly, more inquisitive, and energetic. The young one's temper tantrums are gone. The wife and I are more patient. We are all more optimistic.

"I should also mention a friend of mine who has a grandmother almost a hundred years old. She has intact teeth. She sees and speaks well. She lives in a rural area, walks barefoot to the lands and homestead, and sleeps on an animal hide on the ground in an old-style African hut. She refuses a bed and keeps giving them away when her grandchildren buy them for her."

THE SPIRITUAL CONNECTION

Gabriel Cousens, M.D., Patagonia, Arizona, director of Tree of Life Rejuvenation Center: "I applied Earthing first to myself and my wife. We both felt a difference. Our sleep is deeper. We used to go barefoot some of the time. Now we go barefoot all the time.

"In my work, I am on the go all day long. Now I find myself getting up earlier than before, and despite a half hour or an hour less sleep than I normally used to get, I have more energy. I've always been a high-energy person, but now I have more.

"My clinical impression is that Earthing helps decrease inflammation in people with autoimmune disorders. I have seen it make a difference for people with depression and anxiety. At the Tree of Life Rejuvenation Center, we recommend that everyone who comes here for treatment sleeps on grounding sheets, and everyone benefits in some way or another. People are more relaxed, sleep better, and have more energy as a result.

"Beyond these things, Earthing represents a whole way of thinking. It really speaks to the problem today that people on this planet have lost touch with the Earth and have not returned to the Earth. They have gotten further and further away. From a biblical perspective, people who lose touch with the Earth lose touch with God. There is a whole deeper understanding here. Earthing reconnects us to the Earth, to others, and, in a sense, to God."

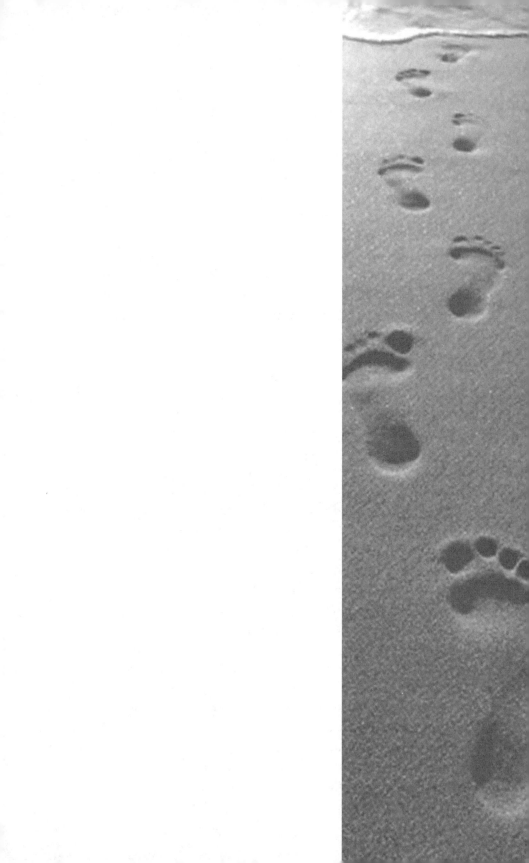

CHAPTER 13

The Feminine Connection: Earthing and Women

Women seem to get it.

They seem to respond intuitively and immediately to the "barefoot connection" and to the healing and energy of Mother Earth. This is not in any way a criticism of the masculine mind, but simply an observation based on years of demonstrating and explaining the concept of Earthing to thousands of people.

"Connect to the Earth and heal" was the way one group of women, in chorus, described Earthing some years ago.

Women seem to enjoy kicking off their shoes at the desk or at home, something you will rarely see a man do. It's not so much that the shoes are uncomfortable, but rather more of a primordial and harmonious connection to the Earth that women may feel more intimately than men.

Women are caregivers by nature. Clint Ober has found that after experiencing the benefits of Earthing, women want to go out and tell everyone in their circle of family and friends. By comparison, men generally want to know how it works.

There is also an appearance factor here. One woman with multiple sclerosis who participated in a one-day Earthing study visited the restroom at the end of the day and then rushed back to the testing center all excited. "I look different," she said. "Like I used to look years ago." Other women have made this comment, even after just a half hour of grounding. And after sleeping grounded for a period of time, women often say they feel better and look better. They say their skin has more radiance, their eyes are brighter, and they have more vitality. The impact on feeling and appearance is likely from a combination of things: elimination of an electron deficiency, better sleep, reduced stress and pain, and more natural and balanced functioning within the body. The feedback suggests that these factors work to help normalize many ongoing health issues and may even be helpful in the struggle against weight gain.

Earthing may contribute on the weight front in part by making you feel more relaxed and normalizing your level of cortisol (the stress hormone). People under stress often have a hard time following a healthy diet. They will frequently eat the wrong things to fill an emotional need or because of lack of time to prepare something healthy for themselves.

The body produces excess cortisol in times of physical and psychological stress. The hormone revs up fat and carbohydrate metabolism for fast energy. Too much stress and too much cortisol in the system can boost the appetite and, according to some studies, promote weight gain. What's more, stress and cortisol can promote fat deposition around the middle, a highly unhealthy and unsightly buildup referred to as abdominal adiposity. The problem with this form of belly fat is that it produces inflammatory chemicals and is a paramount feature of the metabolic syndrome that leads to cardiovascular disease and diabetes. We haven't specifically researched Earthing's effect on weight yet, but quite a few people have remarked about finding it easier to lose weight and keep weight off.

Hormones are a central—and often confusing—concern to women throughout much of their lives. No research has been done to date regarding hormones and Earthing other than a pivotal study on cortisol that we described earlier in Chapter 5. It is well known that hormones work in harmony with each other, even though we are far from understanding all the complex give-and-take and up-and-down interactions. Often, when the body's production of one hormone is off, others are affected, kind of like a domino effect. Cortisol is a close steroid relative of progesterone and more distantly to estrogen. So there could be some impact here that has not been measured yet. Something positive is happening, though. We have received feedback from many women describing relief from debilitating symptoms of PMS and menopause, sometimes quite rapidly.

IN THEIR OWN WORDS

In the original cortisol study published in 2004, the participants provided comments on their health issues prior to and after eight weeks of sleeping grounded. Following is a summary of feedback from five of the female participants. Their responses represent a vision of possibilities from Earthing after just a short period of time. Keep in mind that each person is an individual and is likely to respond differently from the next person. However, the feedback is fairly typical of many other observations made over the years.

Participant No. 1, fifty-three years old, menopausal

Pre-Study Complaints

- Difficulty going to sleep.
- Wakes up two to three times a night for last three years.
- Muscle cramps in legs.
- Chronic muscle pain throughout body.
- Hot flashes.

End of Study Feedback

- "Fall asleep faster and easier."
- "Neck pain lessened."
- "Leg and foot cramps have lessened."
- "Arm and lower back pain gone by the very first week."
- "TMJ (temporomandibular joint disorder) problem significantly improved."
- "Reduction in hot flashes."

Participant No. 2, twenty-four years old

Pre-Study Complaints

- Trouble sleeping for seventeen years; takes a long time to fall asleep; wakes up after several hours and can't sleep again; wakes up exhausted.

- Daily headaches.
- Migraines one week before period.
- Menstrual cramps, mood swings, bloating, irritability, depression, and weight gain.
- Digestion: bloating, nausea, diarrhea, gas, and constipation.

End of Study Feedback

- "By the third night, decreased time to go to sleep and slept through the night."
- "Able to fall back asleep within a few minutes after waking up, and no more nightmares."
- "Wake up refreshed instead of exhausted."
- "No more daily headaches."
- "Decreased PMS, including food cravings, bloating, and depression."
- "Digestion improved with less bloating, constipation, and nausea."

Participant No. 3, fifty-two years old, menopausal

Pre-Study Complaints

- Sleeps very lightly.
- Wakes up feeling tense several times during the night.
- Wakes up feeling tired in morning; feel tired all day.
- Pain in left hip, sporadic for several years.
- Allergies (food and airborne) since age thirteen.
- Digestion: gas.

End of Study Feedback

- "Have felt more rested and feel like I need an hour less sleep per night."
- "Deeper relaxation."
- "Stopped having any pain at all in my left hip."
- "First few days, I experienced tingling and heat in areas of my previous

physical injuries—similar to an acupuncture treatment. After about three days, these vague feelings subsided."

- "Allergies have definitely lessened."

- "Better digestion."

- "I noticed that I stopped clenching my jaw at night."

- The participant reported that her husband, who was not part of the study, but who was sleeping grounded next to her, "began sleeping fewer hours, has more energy, and has stopped snoring."

Participant No. 4, forty-two years old

Pre-Study Complaints

- Trouble falling asleep; light restless sleep.

- Wakes up feeling tired; also, trouble waking up from naps.

- Fibromyalgia since 1992 car accident; a lot of joint pain in arms, legs, ankles.

- Gastrointestinal upset; gas.

End of Study Feedback

- "The general quality of my sleep improved; not immediate, but a gradual change."

- "Sleeping much deeper."

- "A lot less fatigue because of less pain."

- "My fibromyalgia has improved considerably because of diminished pain and fatigue; the joint pain is gone, with occasional pain in the left arm."

- "I am feeling much better, I haven't been sick at all."

Participant No. 5, forty-four years old

Pre-Study Complaints

- Trouble sleeping; wakes up two to three times each night with physical discomfort.

- Numb fingers on left hand for last four months; carpal tunnel syndrome.

- Bad cramps, breast tenderness, mood swings, weight gain, painful heavy periods, and uterine fibroids for many years.

- Hot flashes at night (or maybe night sweats).

- History of anxiety attacks.

End of Study Feedback

- "Gradually sleeping better"

- "Two episodes of waking up between 4:30 and 5:30 AM with anxiety that subsides by early afternoon.

- "Less numbness in hand and fingers, especially at night; not needing to wear a brace at night."

- "Menstrual periods not as severe; cramps not as strong."

- "Feeling better physically and emotionally."

FAST TRACK TO VIBRANT— A ONE-HOUR EARTHING "TIME TRIAL"

How fast can Earthing improve vitality? A 2012 women's wellness conference in Southern California was the setting for an informal experiment to put that question to the test.

About one hundred women in attendance filled out questionnaires before and after a one-hour talk on Earthing. The questions covered individual assessments about energy, pain, stress/irritability, mood, circulation, and flexibility. About half the audience was familiar with Earthing.

The experiment was set up in this way:

Upon entering the hotel conference room, the women received a "goody bag" containing the questionnaire, a pen, an Earthing patch and cord, and a pocket mirror that lights up. Why the mirror? So they could easily view themselves before and after the talk, and see how they looked.

Once seated, the attendees filled out the "before" section of the questionnaire asking for their subjective impressions on how they felt, using a 1 to 10 scale.

Prior to the presentation, an Earthing wiring system had been laid out throughout the room. It allowed each attendee to place the patch on the bottom of one foot, and then connect the cord to the room-wide Earthing system connected to grounded wall outlets.

At the end of the talk, everyone filled out the "after" section of the questionnaire. Here are the questions and the results:

1. ENERGY

   Q: Before (or after) Earthing, my energy level is _____ *(a numerical range from horrible, to OK, to magnificent).*

   A: 78 percent reported more energy, on average an increase of about 40 percent.

2. PAIN

   Q: The level of pain in my body before (or after) Earthing is _____ *(a numerical range from extremely painful, to OK, to I am pain free).*

   A: 60 percent of those with pain said they had less pain at the end, and an average decrease of about 30 percent.

3. STRESS

   Q: My level of stress and irritability before (or after) Earthing is _____ *(a numerical range from terrible, I am extremely stressed, to OK, to I feel calm/centered).*

   A: 77 percent reported less stress, on average about 50 percent better.

4. MOOD

   Q: My overall mood before (or after) Earthing is _____ *(a numerical range from terrible, I feel extremely low, to OK, to my mood is wonderful).*

   A: 82 percent said their mood had improved, with an average of 40 percent.

5. COMPLEXION

   Q: Before (or after) Earthing, when I look into the mirror, my face looks _____ *(a numerical range from dull & pale, to OK, to vibrant & full of color).*

   A: 73 percent thought they looked better, with an average improvement of 38 percent. We attributed the change to improved circulation and more calmness, even from just an hour of Earthing.

6. CIRCULATION

Q: Before (or after) Earthing, the temperature of my hands/feet are _____ (*a numerical range from poor—my hands/feet are ice, to OK, to great—my hands/feet are warm*).

A: 65 percent stated that their circulation had improved, and on average by 32 percent.

7. FLEXIBILITY

Q: Before (or after) Earthing, if I reach down to touch my toes, my flexibility is _____ (*a numerical range from poor, I am extremely stiff, to OK, to excellent, I feel very flexible*).

A: 62 percent reported improvement, with about a 23 percent improvement.

The results were "phenomenal, demonstrating how rapidly Earthing can enhance a woman's vitality, and likely a man's as well, although guys being guys they might be more reluctant to admit it," said Christy Westen, D.C., who gave the talk on Earthing and organized the experiment.

Keep in mind that these changes occurred within an hour of being seated on typically hard, uncomfortable conference chairs next to people you don't know.

Dr. Westen summed up the experience thusly: "Most people think that creating more vitality in life requires a ton of time, effort, and sacrifice. You have to sweat it out in the gym, strenuously try to eat the perfect diet, and offload as much stress as possible. To be sure, these are essential ingredients in a healthy lifestyle recipe, but often not so easy to accomplish. Earthing, on the other hand, requires no strain whatsoever and is, in fact, one of the easiest things you can do for your health. Just reconnect to the Earth, and even in one single hour you can feel a difference, sometimes profoundly, and without any side effects! Make this a routine in your life and you really put yourself on a direct path to becoming simply vibrant!"

STORIES OF MENSTRUAL AND MENOPAUSAL RELIEF

Amanda Ward, N.D., Encinitas, California, naturopathic doctor: "I started Earthing myself and had phenomenal results. My sleep was deeper. When I would become run down, I would wrap myself up in a grounding sheet and recover quickly. However, the most dramatic effect was on my own menstrual issues. I used to have horrific PMS with heavy periods and severe cramping and pain. Nothing I tried was helping me much, even though I have a lot of tools at my disposal as a health practitioner. At times the situation would be debilitating enough so that I had to stay at home.

"After about two months of Earthing, I started to notice an improvement. Then every month my periods would become a little better. In about a year, my menstrual difficulties completely resolved. Now, I might get a bit of irritability, but all the physical symptoms are gone.

"As I began to see the improvements in my own life, I began recommending Earthing to patients. I do a lot of hormone balancing and nutrition to support women's health issues. I use a broad array of methods, so it is hard to say exactly which treatment is helping the most. However, patients have told me that they feel more balanced with Earthing than they do on the other programs alone. My clinical impression is that women who do the Earthing along with bioidentical hormones definitely seem to have a superior experience. There is a lot of synergy here. Hormonal imbalances are so prevalent, and Earthing seems to be such a simple and profound tool to smooth out those imbalances.

"I have seen particularly good results with perimenopause and menopause, with reduction of symptoms like hot flashes, night sweats, insomnia, and irritability.

"Some of the mothers in my practice have told me that they have used Earthing sheets and helped their kids recover faster from cold and flu symptoms. I've heard this feedback even from women whose children have weaker immune systems and tend to be sick frequently. The mothers will take the grounding sheet they themselves use and wrap up the kids in it when they are watching TV. If the kids sleep grounded, I've heard, they sleep a lot better."

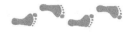

Dale Teplitz, M.A., San Diego, California, health researcher: "Ever since my periods began at age thirteen, and until I was forty-five, I suffered routinely with severe PMS and menstrual symptoms. In the week prior to each period, I experienced gradually increasing water retention, food cravings, headaches, and weight gain. I was irritable. My skin was itchy and uncomfortable. My body ached and felt painful to the touch. For several nights prior to every period, I could not sleep. Over the years, I took diuretics to help with the water retention and sleeping pills for those difficult nights.

"PMS also affected my personality and relationships; I had emotional ups and downs, anxiety, and often felt depressed. Medication left me feeling emotionally numb.

"Once my period began, the PMS symptoms would go away to be replaced by severe cramps and heavy bleeding. The pain and fatigue often prevented me from working. I lived on anti-inflammatories during this time, which disturbed my digestion.

"At the age of forty-five, I started sleeping grounded. One month later, all my PMS symptoms went away. I was astounded. In one stroke, I was able to eliminate the sleeping pills, diuretics, anti-inflammatories, and other medications. I was free of symptoms, and I felt like a new person.

"Two years later, I entered menopause. I was feeling a bit anxious about what might lie ahead because I had heard horror stories from other women. It seemed that those who had a lot of PMS issues had the most difficulty going through menopause.

"To my surprise, I sailed into menopause effortlessly. I had a gradual decrease in the frequency and duration of periods until they eventually disappeared. I did not experience sleeplessness. I only had mild and brief hot flashes, which I determined were related to certain foods or red wine. There were no hormonal-type mood swings all my friends reported. Some of my friends have had menopause symptoms for more than ten years now, well into their sixties.

"Another thing that amazes me is that when I was in my early forties, I had been diagnosed with osteopenia, a condition in which bone density is below normal and may lead to osteoporosis. For several years in a row, I had a dual energy x-ray absorptionmetry scan, or DEXA scan, that showed decreased density of my thigh and ankle bones. When I was tested again at age forty-eight, after sleeping grounded for three years, the osteopenia was gone. I was tested again at fifty-two, and it was still gone! My bone density looked great.

"I am convinced that Earthing took away my symptoms of PMS, cramps, and menopause. I doubt that indigenous women who live directly on the Earth are troubled with symptoms of hormone imbalance. I can't imagine how much better my life would have been if I had learned about Earthing thirty years sooner, but nobody knew about it then. So I consider myself lucky to have heard about it at all. I could have continued suffering much longer."

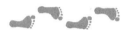

Melissa Dawahare, N.D., R.N., Tempe, Arizona, naturopathic physician: "Prior to starting Earthing in 2012, I routinely experienced moderate menstrual cramping (at a 3 to 4 level out of 10). That stopped with Earthing, and right away.

"I have found that I recover from intense cardio and resistance workouts faster, with no or minimal muscle soreness. Before, there was always some discomfort afterward.

"I noticed that my immune system appears to be stronger. I don't catch a cold as easy and if I feel like I am coming down with one, sleeping grounded takes it away.

"My kids sleep grounded as well. They also have better immunity. Their colds are less severe and they last half the time. They sleep longer, harder, and deeper."

"I HAVE MY HEALTH BACK"

Elizabeth Hughes, Ph.D., Madison County, Wisconsin, former corporate executive: "At age twenty-one, I developed fever, sore throat, muscle soreness, headaches, swollen glands, and fatigue. My doctor thought I had a case of mononucleosis, a viral condition that frequently strikes young adults. I spent a lot of time in bed and out of commission for the next twenty-five or so years, with one variation or another of some sickness. It seemed to me that my doctors used different names for the shifting symptoms according to whatever mystery disease was in vogue at the time: things like chronic fatigue, Epstein-Barr virus, fibromyalgia, and Ramsay Hunt syndrome. One doctor thought I had MS. I didn't.

"I was stuck in a system where doctors have great intentions but few explanations about how you got sick and very little to heal you with. A few doctors said it was all in my head and offered antidepressants and psychotherapy. Early on a team of six interns reviewed my case and said they didn't know what was wrong even though my symptoms were obvious.

"Many chemicals made me sick. For a long time, I couldn't set foot in a hairdresser's salon or department store. New synthetic fabrics, carpets, outgassing solvents, and volatile compounds were a problem.

"I did all I could to get well. When conventional treatments failed, I tried the alternatives. I drank 16 ounces of wheat grass juice daily to detoxify myself. I ate pure organic uncooked food. I had my amalgam fillings removed to get rid of mercury in my body. I got some temporary relief from all these things, but nothing lasting or really substantial.

"Despite ongoing health issues, I managed to earn a Ph.D. and work in corporate America at a very high level. When I got very sick, I just had to go on disability and drop out for a while.

"I was always searching for an answer, but I could not find it. I even joined support groups with other women who had the same kind of complaints. It was so bad and so hopeless for some of those women that they actually talked about committing suicide. After some temporary relief from one thing or another, I would go back to work so I could earn enough money to pay for treating the next episode.

"Around 2005, I learned about Earthing and got grounded. Within six weeks, I was a new person. I was amazed. Shocked is actually a better word. There was no more pain in my body. My symptoms of whatever the doctors variably called my condition were gone, as were the tender, painful breasts, something I had always dealt with during menstruation. Later, the hot flashes I began experiencing as I entered menopause subsided and then disappeared with additional Earthing.

"I got my health back, and without any medication. And it's been that way now for eight years."

MOTHER EARTH HELPING MOTHERS

Return to Dancing After Childbirth, Knee Pain

Olivia Biera, Los Angeles, California, healing arts consultant: "I've been involved for years professionally as a traditional Aztec dancer, performing at festivals and historical locations. This is very vigorous dancing, very lower-body intensive. After having my daughter in 2005, I was anxious to get back into it, but I didn't have the same flexibility and muscularity that I had had before. I think I pushed myself too hard trying to come back and did something to my right knee that caused chronic inflammation. An MRI showed no tear, just deep inflammation. The knee was like one big swollen balloon that hurt badly. It was difficult to walk up stairs. Driving and carrying my baby made it worse. In addition, my right hip was also giving me a lot of trouble after childbirth.

"I had to do something. Massage and other therapies I tried weren't working. It was almost impossible to stretch. At one point in 2007, I was two weeks away from exploratory knee surgery. That's when I started sleeping and working grounded. I immediately noticed an ability to sleep through the pain. From one week to the next, the inflammation began to go down. After about six weeks, it was 30 to 40 percent less—and that was without icing. Simply sleeping well and using essential oils for relief. I no longer needed to sleep with a pillow between my legs to ease the pain. The pain was slipping away. I never had that surgery. Today, in 2013, I continue to sleep grounded. My knee is 100 percent!

"Perhaps the biggest surprise is what happened to my nicotine craving. No matter how many good health practices I followed, like yoga and good diet, I couldn't kick the craving. I'd been smoking for thirteen years when I became pregnant. I quit. It's not that I smoked a lot, but at the end of my workday I had a craving for cigarettes that would drive me nuts. I would smoke one cigarette and then maybe another cigarette. After six weeks, the craving was gone, and I haven't smoked since.

"I also experienced a definite release of emotional stresses. At the time I started grounding, I had a lot going on in my life. I definitely noticed right off the bat a sense of rejuvenation and emotional 'grounding.' I was grounded physically and that grounded me emotionally and even spiritually, in the sense of being connected to the Earth.

"My sleep pattern changed as well. I recognized quickly that I was sleeping deeper. I also noticed something with my daughter that was quite interesting. She always used to fall asleep in a curled, fetal position. She would typically roll around the bed until she found the perfect curved position to sleep in. Then, at age two, when she started to sleep grounded, she fell asleep straight as a board—the very first night. It was like a magnet pulled her into the sheets, and she slept totally relaxed. She is eight now and a very deep sleeper. I sense it strongly when she becomes overly 'amped' from electronics, and then irritable and unable to relax before bed. It is a relief to be able to use the Earthing sheet.

"At my office, we use grounded floor mats. There are computers, printers, telephones, and electronic equipment, which probably emit a lot of electromagnetic pollution. I myself used to get tired. Not after I began working grounded. I grounded the whole office and there has been a tremendous increase in productivity and in terms of being alert, not having computer drain, staying with the game, and getting it done."

Single Mom and Son Sleeping and Coping Better

Donna Zerger, Colorado Springs, civil engineer–math teacher: "Earthing has had major benefits for me and my son since we started sleeping grounded in early 2013.

"Personally, I sleep so much better and deeper and notice that I dream again. I have a renewed sense of calmness that extends into my days and work world and makes it easier for me to cope and separate myself from other people's 'stuff.' My energy level has increased dramatically and I have more focus. Earthing has reduced, and made nearly nonexistent, many years of neck pain due to two vertebras being fused together. My hot flashes are half of what they were before, so that's another factor in improved sleep. And my skin is not as dry as before. It's much smoother. At one point, a week after I started grounding, I was putting in very long work weeks at the school and people were remarking how well rested and younger I looked!

"My twelve-year-old son is experiencing deeper sleep, more vivid dreams, and a much better sense of well-being and calmness. He has dyslexia, dysgraphia, dyscalculia, focus issues, bad gut, and wheat/gluten intolerance, but since we've been grounding we have seen school grades, moods, coping skills, and reaction to food greatly improved. Since he is sleeping better, it is easier for him to get up for school. That goes for me as well. And we're both staying calmer and having an easier time dealing with conflict. This is a profound benefit.

"Another mom we know whose son has autistic-type issues has noticed improvements since starting Earthing well.

"And then there are the animals in our lives: one dog and three cats. I have the half sheet horizontal across the bottom of the bed and it is quite common to wake in the night and/or morning to find that the cats have burrowed beneath the blankets to gain access to the sheet. The cats will also sit or lay on our Earthing mats at our computers. Our dog also sneaks onto the bed to lay on the sheet, and especially sought it out recently when he hurt his hind leg. It seems that our animals want to get grounded and fully 'charged.'"

Pregnancy Boost

Stephanie Okeafor, Paradise Valley, Arizona, personal trainer and microcurrent therapist: "The most dramatic thing for me has been the effect on my pregnancy, and particularly the first trimester. This was my first pregnancy.

"I am a very active person and follow a rigorous fitness routine. When I became pregnant, I didn't run as much, but I was still doing the same intensity of lifting, lunges, and cross-training activities. I realized quickly that I was okay in the moment doing these workouts, but afterward— within the next hour or so—I would feel pretty exhausted.

"I would go home and say okay, I'm pregnant, I'll take a nap. I need to take care of myself. But I never really needed a big nap. I would lie down on the grounding sheet, and after twenty minutes I would get up, feeling completely alert and rested, and ready to go.

"I have had a very easy pregnancy compared to most women I've talked to. No sickness at all. I worked out the entire time. I had excellent energy except for after the workouts. Also, it was over 100 degrees every day for the last half of my pregnancy. People wondered how I did so well with all the heat.

Is There an Earthing-Fertility Connection?

Russell Whitten, D.C., Santa Barbara, California, chiropractor: "I started grounding patients back in 2000, and I had some great feedback from many of them. A few told me, however, they didn't know if it was working or not. I began to realize they no longer had pain and had forgotten they had it before, unless I mentioned it.

"My patients have frequently told me that their dreams become more vivid when they start to sleep grounded and, in some cases, almost psychedelic-like.

"Perhaps the most amazing Earthing story I have witnessed involves my own wife, Joey. She had not been able to get pregnant during the eight years of her first marriage. Then, for the first six years of our relationship, she was still unable to conceive. From a medical standpoint, everything appeared normal, but it just never happened. In 2000, we started sleeping grounded, and within a month she became pregnant, for the first time, at the age of thirty-five.

"In my opinion, there was nothing else but grounding that could explain it. I had been giving her chiropractic adjustments for a couple of years at that point so that wasn't what made the difference.

"Within six months of meeting Clint Ober, I had grounded roughly fifty of my patients' beds. It was soon reported back to me that several of my patients who were in their forties had become pregnant after starting to sleep grounded. Each had had their children in their twenties and now years later were able to conceive again. It seemed like more than just a coincidence to me. I also heard that women's periods became less symptomatic and their hormonal systems seemed to normalize. There may be great potential here for the fertility industry.

"Joey gave birth in April 2001 to a boy. He was born at home on our grounded bed. We named him Tiger because my wife had had a vivid dream while pregnant that she had a tiger in her belly. We wanted to create a name that said something about him and his spirit."

"I'm absolutely sure that being fit helps the situation. Conceiving when you're in good shape puts you ahead in the game compared to someone who starts out her pregnancy not in shape. However, I have a lot of friends who are in great shape, and they've had a hard time throughout their pregnancy. I know each pregnancy is different, but getting great sleep and grounding for an extra twenty minutes here and there during the day I'm sure is a big reason for my energy level."

Note: Stephanie had a home birth in October 2009. The rest of her story was filled in by her husband Chike, a retired professional football player: "It all went beautifully. Stephanie rocketed through it. She was very powerful. I was awestruck. Our midwife was very impressed. I was able to catch my daughter and cut the umbilical cord. She came out and her eyes were clear and alert. She started feeding pretty much right away. Stephanie is six foot and I am six foot five, and Anaya Louise, our daughter, weighed in at 10 pounds, 4 ounces. Mother and baby did very well, and both are staying grounded."

In early 2014, Stephanie reported that she was about to give birth a third time. Her second pregnancy had been a breeze, she said. Now, even having to deal with a healthy and active four-year-old daughter and a two-year-old son (meaning very little nap time), the third pregnancy had nevertheless been easy for her as she neared the end. She, her husband, and the kids, stay consistently grounded. "I know it's made a big difference for all of us," she said.

Rx For Pregnancy Hives

U.S. doctors call it pruritic urticarial papules and plaques of pregnancy (PUPPP) and European doctors, polymorphic eruption of pregnancy (PEP). In simple language, it is an outbreak of annoying, itchy hives on the body that occurs during the third trimester in about 1 out of 160 pregnancies. The condition has no known cause, although some research says it may be due to maternal hypertension.

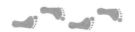

Jasmin White, Rochester Hills, Michigan, community mental health counselor: "When I was pregnant with my first daughter, I had pregnancy hives for fourteen weeks. Nothing got rid of them. It was horrible. When I was carrying my second child, I developed the hives again, but much later, at thirty-two weeks, and they were much worse. My doctors tried different medication, but nothing worked. My husband was using an Earthing sheet and it occured to me at that point to give it a try. I'm so glad I did! I slept on the sheet for two days and the hives were gone! It was amazing. I slept on it the rest of my pregnancy and will do so again the next time I have a child. It saved my sanity. For sure, I will be sleeping on the sheet for every pregnancy I go through in the future.

"We share the sheet with our kids (ages two and four) whenever they develop eczema outbreaks, which is frequent. It seems to clear up the eczema quickly, as quickly as one night of use. We also keep them on the sheet when they are sick and it seems to help them get better quicker."

CHAPTER 14

The Sports Connection: Earthing in Action

Biophysicist James Oschman tells the story of a friend who ran in a marathon. Part of the way through the race, he developed a very painful blister on his foot, yanked off his shoes, and pushed on without them. Not only was he able to finish the race without pain, he was also very surprised at the end to find that his blister was completely gone.

If that seems hard to believe, consider the most dramatic application of Earthing: the experience of competitors at cycling's premier event, the Tour de France. The success of grounding in one of the most challenging races in the world is extraordinary.

The grounding-cycling story starts in 2003, when Jeff Spencer, D.C., a prominent sports medicine specialist based in Pasadena, California, contacted Clint Ober. He had heard about Earthing from a San Diego doctor and was intrigued by the concept. Dr. Spencer, a former Olympic cyclist, works with elite athletes functioning at the highest level of performance and applies cutting-edge methods to support optimum health and enhance recovery from exertion and injury. This was his assignment during five Tour de France competitions. During four of them, 2003 to 2005, and again in 2007, he utilized Earthing.

Here's his story.

EARTHING AT THE TOUR DE FRANCE

"I've had the good fortune of working with many athletes at the highest level in terms of getting them to the top of their game and keeping them there. You can't imagine what a challenge that is when the sports event is the Tour de France. My No. 1 job was to make sure that the riders showed up every day, at the starting line, 100 percent mentally and physically ready for the rides of their lives. On the other side of that was to make sure that we had very aggressive recovery strategies so that they could survive this inhumane event called the Tour de France. In doing so, I had to develop as compressed a time line for injury and full-body recovery as possible. The challenge gave me tremendous flexibility in putting together a 'tool kit' that would give us a competitive advantage. In the Tours that I worked, we lost only four riders—one to a broken arm, one to severe tendonitis, another to a broken arm, and the other to a broken hand. Otherwise, all the other riders finished, which is really unheard of in this sport.

"As a doctor who has worked with some of the best of the best in the sports world, I've found that it's essential to never allow yourself to believe that what you did before is any guarantee of future success. So, by definition, I'm always looking for new innovations that will take me to the

"Le Tour Terrible"

The Tour de France is among the most brutal athletic events in the world—comparable to running three marathons a day for twenty-one straight days. Racers may climb as much as a total of 30,000 feet in a single day's stage. That's six miles straight up. The race covers 2,100 miles on the ground and ranges from sea level to 8,700 feet.

In July, when the race is run, the weather is very hot in France. The narrow asphalt roads over which the Tour is run start to crack, blister, and soften, making the going extremely treacherous. Falling on that kind of surface is like landing on a cheese grater. Cyclists suffer massive abrasions affectionately known as "road rash."

The traffic around the racers as they go from stage to stage is intense. There are more than 170 cyclists racing in a very crowded pack. They are shadowed by a chaotic convoy of support vehicles carrying mechanics, spare bicycles and parts, as well as vehicles with Tour officials, media, and security personnel. The combination of cyclists, high speeds, narrow roads, cars, and motorcycles is a recipe for mishaps. Crashes are common and can cause serious physical trauma.

next level and give me that competitive edge over the competition. I am continually remodeling my ultimate clinical 'tool box' so as to stay current with state-of-the-art equipment and methods.

"When I first heard about Earthing, it sounded very interesting to me. I had never heard of it before, but it sounded like something that might be useful for what I do. I contacted the developer of the technology (Clint Ober) and asked to meet with him. When we talked, it became clear to me that if Earthing did what he said it was supposed to do, it could give the Tour cyclists a tremendous advantage.

"Earthing wouldn't change anything I normally did. And all somebody had to do is lay down and go to sleep or relax like they would normally do. This would help them sleep and relax, so I was told. This was very appealing. I knew that when I would spend time outdoors with my feet in the sand or I'd walk at the beach with my feet close to the water, I would feel a lot better.

"But I first had to try the technology on myself. I was not willing to use anything for my patients that I didn't know worked from my own firsthand experience. For about five years, I had been suffering with the consequences of mercury poisoning. At one point, my health was quite debilitated. I had been receiving treatment for it and was improving gradually. I was getting better. But after grounding myself one night, I felt a significant improvement. When I awoke the next morning, I felt much better. I had more energy. I had had difficulty concentrating before, but now I had greater clarity of thinking. I had less pain. Less irritability. My body felt like it had been washed from inside out. After three or four nights of sleeping better and feeling better, I knew that this was something for real. I recognized that this is something that could have tremendous value not just for me but also for my patients and the cyclists at the Tour de France.

"I was, to say the least, impressed. I asked Clint if he could create a prototype system for me to take and use at the Tour de France. The challenge is that the Tour is so difficult mentally and physically that the riders have a hard time sleeping. And if you don't sleep, you don't recover. If you don't recover, the body breaks down, the mind goes down, and you can unnecessarily get injured or sick, which is catastrophic for a top Tour effort."

A Huge Difference

"Clint agreed and came up with a prototype system. It had a metallic snap at one end that connected to a wire that ran to an outside ground rod. Clint handmade all the wiring and taught me how to use the system. It was ready just in time for the 2003 Tour de France. And it made a huge difference. The severe mental and physical strain from daily competition needs to be discharged from the body while the rider is relaxing and recovering, so we need technology available at night in order that the rider gets up the next morning fully recovered.

"I saw the same experiences among the riders that I had experienced myself. They slept much better. And that's a big deal in a competition like this where cyclists have a very hard time sleeping because they are so overstimulated from the Tour's intensity and, ironically, often overtired. When they can't rest and sleep enough, they can break down. When trying to sustain high performance at this level, team physicians always wonder how they can improve sleep and take advantage of the sleep downtime. So Earthing was like an answer to my prayers. The riders reported less mental tension and stress. They felt calmer. Their decision-making was good. Their vitality and morale were really high."

Accelerated Healing

"We also applied Earthing, along with other treatments, to accelerate tissue repair and wound healing from injuries sustained during the competition. The results were phenomenal. The cyclists recovered much faster.

"The most dramatic case involved a cyclist in the 2005 Tour who suffered severe lacerations to his upper right arm after crashing through the rear window of a support car that had stopped abruptly (see Figure 14-1 on the opposite page). He managed to make it to the finish line. He immediately received aggressive medical treatment and was taken to a local hospital for stitches. When I saw him on the team bus right after that day's Tour stage, he had shock written all over his face. His jersey and riding shorts were bloody. His arm had been tightly bandaged to stop the bleeding. When the bandages were removed, you could actually see the tendons and bones through the torn flesh. It looked like somebody had chopped up his arm with a carving knife. Later at the hotel, we saw extensive stitches in his upper arm, as well as his elbow, hand, and chin. He had a large purple bruise on his leg, as if someone had hit him with a lead pipe. The team had serious reservations about whether

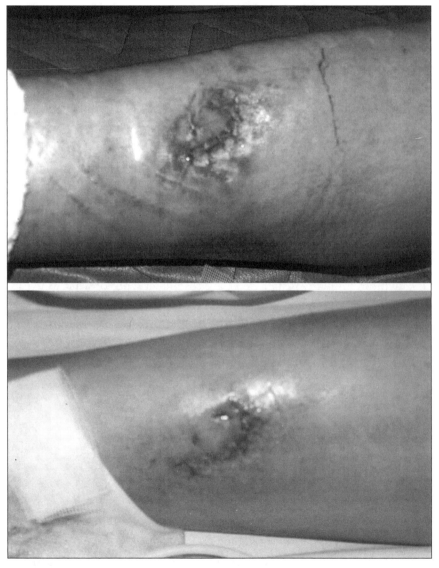

Figure 14-1. Rapid wound healing. Overnight grounding accelerated the healing of this, and many other similar cycling wounds. (*Photos courtesy of Jeff Spencer, D.C.*)

he could continue in the Tour because of the extent of his injuries. Everybody doubted he would be able to return to competition the next day.

"I asked for twelve hours—basically overnight—to try to help him heal enough to continue racing. I knew that Earthing could make a big difference. Everybody agreed it was worth a shot as long as he wasn't in danger of hurting himself further. So I applied multiple grounded electrodes to his arm and leg and he slept grounded that night, as he had throughout the competition. When he awoke the next day, there wasn't nearly the pain, redness, soreness, or swelling he had the night before. He didn't seem nearly as bad off as would be normally expected. He felt up to going out that day and racing. Our high hopes were that he could continue, finish the day's ride, and get stronger and heal more each subsequent day. I took the patches off him and gave him additional care with other techniques. I taped up his bruised leg, and he was rebandaged, and off he went to race that day's stage. It turned out that he was indeed able to put in a full day's ride and perform his role for the team. The other cyclists were overjoyed. He ultimately finished the competition and contributed to the team victory. To an outsider, his recovery was nothing less than miraculous.

"In my experience with Earthing, this kind of response is not surprising anymore. In many instances, I have seen an absence of what we regard as a normal inflammatory response. When individuals are grounded, injuries lack much—and I mean much—of the typical degree of pain and redness. Tissue repair is accelerated.

"At the end of the 2005 Tour, the team director asked me about the condition of the riders.

" 'They're doing great,' I said.

" 'What about tendonitis?' he asked. Cyclists have a high incidence of tendon inflammation in their legs because of the prolonged and intense strain they put themselves through.

" 'It wasn't a problem,' I said.

" 'Anybody sick?' he asked.

" 'No, everybody's good,' I answered.

"He shrugged and said, 'incredible.'

"Acute traumatic injury is common in the world of athletics, so Earthing is a great boon. Grounding helps minimize injury downtime and speed recovery. I know how long it takes to recover normally. And I also know what

Earthing vs. Icing for Injuries— Jeff Spencer's Perspective

"From many years of experience treating the injuries of athletes, I find that Earthing offers healing benefits above and beyond the results we typically see with icing. The classic signs and consequences of injury are much less pronounced, and in some cases don't even develop when I apply Earthing to an injury. The signs are redness, heat, swelling, pain, and decreased range of motion.

"Regardless of the extent of the injury, pain reduction is significant with Earthing compared to ice; frequently, 40 or 50 percent less. I have never experienced that kind of healing with icing. Recovery time is significantly reduced.

"My typical strategy is to apply an Earthing patch on the skin—over or adjacent to the injury site—and then a second patch to a primary acupuncture point on the same side of the body. That means the palm of a hand, if the injury is above the waist, or to the K1 point on the bottom of the foot for an injury to the lower extremities.

"Often, I will apply additional patches on or around the site of an injury. I've used as many as a dozen patches over an injury covering a large area.

"The combination works magically: the sooner after an injury that you apply the patches and the more continuous the care, the faster the recovery. With Earthing, you also have an ideal situation where you can go to sleep with the patches applied to the injury area and get continuous treatment. For added effect, you also can use other Earthing products, like an Earthing mat or sheet.

"I have used Earthing as part of my treatment strategy for several hundred athletes competing at the highest level in different sports for more than ten years. The injuries include abrasions, strains and sprains, wound and postsurgical situations, and recovery from fractures after orthopedic treatment.

"Individuals can apply this technique for themselves, however, they should always seek proper evaluation first from a health professional following any injury. Earthing can be added to the recommended recovery program."

happens when an athlete is grounded. The changes in terms of body recovery from day to day, the ability to repair tissue, to recover from activity and the stresses and strains of the day, are amazing. To me, it's obvious that any athlete should make Earthing part of his or her regular wellness program.

"Earthing also appears to accelerate recovery from surgery, which, as far as the body is concerned, is basically a form of traumatic injury. One of my patients is a champion in Supercross, a wild and wooly sport where off-road motorcycles race in stadium dirt tracks filled with steep jumps and obstacles. My patient suffered a bad shoulder injury that required surgery. He was treated in a variety of ways to speed the healing process, including sleeping grounded. In three weeks, he was able to compete in a national event and win the competition. He made an amazingly rapid recovery."

Less Pain

"Among the different athletes I help, the common feedback I hear about Earthing goes something like this: 'I'm sleeping so much better and have less pain. I get up the next day, and I feel so much more recovered. I can't believe the workouts that I'm doing. I should be more tired. My results and improvement are increasing with more frequency. They're staying at a high level. It takes less effort to get and stay where I am.'

"Athletes say frequently they are able to push through the day better. They don't have that midafternoon energy drop. They get up in the morning with much more clarity, ready to seize the opportunity of the day. They seem to need less sleep. They have better quality of sleep. They may have been used to having eight hours of sleep before. Now they need maybe an hour or so less, but they still can perform at the same level. Matter of fact, they even feel better.

"Professional football players live with one degree or another of pain from all the hard physical contact in their sport. They tell me they just don't have the normal pain that they think they should based on what they do. These are the things that I constantly hear.

"Probably the greatest value that I've found with Earthing is that it provides a rock solid biological platform, a basis, for all the other treatments and care that I use. It makes everything else work so much better. Everybody wants a treatment for a specific problem. Earthing, though, is like a universal antidote. It seems to reset the physiological playing field, allowing the body to be its own best healer and do the job it's designed to do —repair and regenerate itself, and create energy to sustain a long and productive life. I think of Earthing as the primer for a canvas on which I paint all the strategies for getting my clients to the top and keeping them there. In art, if you don't properly prime the canvas, the paint won't stick.

"It's now been more than ten years that I've been Earthing personally and in my work. During that time, there have been only a handful of days that I have not been grounded. On those occasions where for some reason I either forgot my bed pad or the building that I was in didn't allow me to use the technology, I could definitely tell the difference in terms of how I felt and recovered from exercise. I do a lot of traveling, both domestically and internationally, and one of the personal benefits that I found is the dramatic reduction in jet lag. I get up the next day and function fully in the time zone I'm at and not where I came from.

"Earthing is amazingly simple. It's as easy as going barefoot on the beach or in your yard. Or if you have an Earthing device, all you do is plug it in. You lie down, you go to sleep. You do what you normally do. No refills. No prescriptions. No calibrations, settings, timers, no nothing.

"In my view, biology is biology. It doesn't matter who you are. We all share the same basic human biology. What I've observed with high performers in terms of the response to the Earth is exactly what I have observed with patients who aren't athletes. All of us need to perform as best as we can in life and have the stamina to carry out our daily routines, which often are very demanding and stressful. Whatever we can do to enhance our performance and bolster our recovery from day-to-day stresses helps ensure that we become consistent top performers in whatever we do in our lives. That's really what life is all about."

LESS PROTEIN/MUSCLE BREAKDOWN = FASTER RECOVERY

In Chapter 8 we presented a 2010 study showing how Earthing speeds recovery from exercise-induced inflammation involved in common delayed onset muscle soreness (DOMS). In 2013, a group of Polish researchers provided more striking evidence of Earthing's dramatic effect on recovery by measuring blood urea, an indicator of muscle and protein breakdown, before, during, and after exercise on a stationary bicycle.

The results revealed that grounding during exercise significantly lowers urea levels either through liver or kidney processes and generates a positive protein (nitrogen) balance. The findings represent an important benefit for training athletes whose goal is to maintain or increase muscle mass.

The new study involved a double-blind crossover design with forty-two healthy male students from the University of Physical Education and Sport in Gdansk. The participants were divided into two groups and performed two once-a-week exercise stints lasting thirty minutes on a bicycle ergometer; one time while being grounded and one time ungrounded, and at a maximum of half their oxygen intake. Following the exercise they rested for forty minutes. The participants were either grounded or sham grounded via an ankle strap and cord connected to a switch box and then to a metal plumbing pipe. The participants didn't know if the switch was on or off.

"Our study shows that urea concentrations are lower in subjects who are Earthed during physical exercise and recovery compared with the same subjects who are not Earthed," said neurosurgeon Pawel Sokal, M.D., Ph.D., the lead researcher. "Contact with the Earth may have an important effect on human health in rest and exercise, particularly for training athletes. Earthing during exercise prevents protein degradation and thus helps to sustain a positive nitrogen balance."

Dr. Sokal, involved in Earthing research for more than twenty years, believes strongly that grounding affects protein metabolism or/and renal function. "Perhaps alterations in pH from Earthing change the intensity of the urea cycle or even change nitrogen balance and in that way lowers nitrogen breakdown, or promotes urea excretion in kidneys. Further research will clarify this." Urea is the chief nitrogenous waste of mammals and mostly derives from a breakdown of protein (amino acids).

Jeff Spencer, D.C., who has been Earthing athletes for more than a decade, explains that a positive balance with exercise "means that the protein and muscle mass is not being pulverized as occurs normally. Breakdown is less; the body is able to repair better.

"This is a massive effect. It indicates that you can train and work harder and longer. Risk is greatly reduced. Career longevity is improved.

"Every athlete wants to improve performance capacity and longevity, and this study helps explain what I see with athletes who are grounded. They are training harder, better, getting more benefits, and have faster recovery, and they get more athletic longevity. If you can limit tissue breakdown and accelerate protein synthesis that means more protein creation and better repair.

"But this isn't just for athletes. It's for everybody, whether you are in sports, business, or the everyday stage of life. This is universally applied biology that translates to increased performance, less recovery requirement, and longevity."

Dick Brown, Ph.D., the well-known Oregon exercise physiologist who conducted the earlier Earthing experiment on DOMS, added that "this study shows again that grounding has a positive effect on the body and reinforces the validity of body changes due to grounding. If protein degradation can be reduced while doing exercises as shown here, then grounding can prevent further degradation during recovery."

The study brings up the issue of finding ways to be grounded during exercise. Some types of exercise and training can be conducted outdoors barefoot, or done on conductive mats while barefoot in gyms or on exercise equipment outfitted with grounding access. The study also raises the prospect, as Dr. Sokal notes, that there may be "quite shocking differences" in protein breakdown or altered kidney excretion between barefoot runners and those using running footwear.

EARTHING AND FOOTBALL

Chike Okeafor, former National Football League player: "I've been sleeping grounded regularly for almost a decade after experiencing the effect of grounding on a leg injury. It was a hamstring injury in the back of my knee, plus some deep bruising of the thigh, incurred during a practice session. As I lay on a grounded sheet, I watched a computer monitor connected to a real-time thermal imaging camera. I was amazed to see the colors depicting the intensity of the inflammation from the injury cool down quickly, like within fifteen minutes. The intensity was dramatically different within an hour or so. I felt the difference physically, but to see the changes like that so rapidly was mind-blowing.

"I needed to play that weekend in a big game and there wasn't much time to recover. We were thinking it was going to be nothing short of a miracle to get me ready. My naturopath did some work on me, and I slept grounded the rest of that week. I recovered enough to where I was able to play and without injuring myself further. I was sold on grounding from then on.

"There haven't been very many occasions since then that I do not sleep grounded. I can always feel the difference. In those situations, I always notice that I'm not getting as restful sleep as I do when I am grounded. I used to be a guy who needed eight hours of sleep, and I would take ten if I had the opportunity. I quickly saw that with grounding I was well rested with six hours.

"I also felt a big difference on the days after games. Normally, you are super sore the day after because of the physical nature of the game, from all the hits and banging that goes on. But I learned that grounding the night after a game so dramatically reduced my inflammation that I wasn't nearly as sore. It felt almost as if I skipped that tough day of normal recovery. With grounding, the experience was more like how I used to feel on day two after a game."

EARTHING ON THE TRIATHLETE FRONT

Chris Lieto has won three Ironman titles, the U.S. national title, and finished three times in the top ten at triathlon world championship competitions: "When I first got involved in the sport, I set a goal of being a champion. To reach that goal, I needed to learn how to maximize everything—effort, equipment, food, water, supplements, and my recovery process from injuries and exhaustion.

"Training has always been a big part of the effort. I've always loved it, and enjoyed being outside and healthy. Training is a little different every day, depending on what race is coming up. The Ironman involves a 2.4-mile swim, followed by a 112-mile bike ride, and then when you're done with all that, you run a marathon. That's 26.2 miles. That's a very long and tough day to say the least. But that's just in the Ironman. There are also half-Ironman distances, and other variations on the theme as well.

"Training for me has involved three to eight hours daily on a regular basis, about twenty to twenty-six hours a week total. That includes swimming and biking four or five days a week and running about five or six days a week. There are days of rest and no training at all. When preparing for an Ironman competition, during the course of a week I'll swim probably twelve miles, bike up to fifteen miles, and build up to about eighty miles a week running.

"The sport is tough on your body. You have to train so much and for different activities. This is different from most any other sport. For most sports, you go out and train specifically for one event or one thing, and you train for two to four hours a day. Here, you really put your body through the ringer every day. So recovery is a major issue. Anyone can go out and train. But if you don't have that recovery, and your body's not adapting, then the training is going to hurt you instead of help you. You have to take the time and the focus to recover. You need good sleep and get enough good foods and protein and calories in you. You have to stay on top of everything.

"I've been sleeping grounded for more than eight years, and it has always been a huge boost for my recovery process. I've been able to come back a lot stronger and feel a lot better. I noticed right away that I wouldn't get as fatigued on a daily basis and would be able to work out the next day. You want to get in the workouts day in and day out. But you want to make sure that you recover enough to get that workout to be of benefit. So for me, grounding has been a simple way to recover without really doing anything different.

"During the day, if I have a chance, I'll put my feet on a grounding mat. When I get done with a workout, I make my recovery food and drink, sit down, and wrap my legs in a recovery bag. Any time for me to be hooked into the Earth is good.

"If I have really sore shin splints or a sore calf or a hurting hip, I'll attach a grounded electrode patch right on the spot. The Earth's energy gets fed straight into that point, and the swelling in that area will go down. Once I had an ankle that flared up. For a week, I applied alternate ice and heat, but the swelling wouldn't go away. I put the patch on it, and the following day it felt normal and I was able to run. So I learned to use the patch directly on the spot whenever something feels sore or swollen. I'll put a patch on and I'm good.

"Today, at forty-one, I dedicate much of my energy to Morethansport.org, an organization that develops ways for athletes and athletic events to contribute to local charities and community projects. I don't race as much as I used to, but when I do, I still maintain a high fitness and competitive ability against guys many years younger. Grounding has been a big help in allowing me to do that."

EARTHING AND GOLF LONGEVITY

Ted Barnett, Palm Desert, California, retired mattress factory owner:
"My wife and I owned a mom-and-pop mattress factory. We did at least half the work ourselves and had one or two employees. We made mattresses, delivered them, and set them up in the homes of our customers. In our factory, I was the 'closer.' I ran the big tape-edge machine, which is one of the toughest jobs in a bedding plant. This operation is where you sew the top quilted mattress panel to the side border. People who run this machine for any length of time have problems with their hands because they are constantly pulling hard with their fingers. My hands were in pretty bad shape. I had arthritis, and I was concerned.

"Our factory made some of the first Earthing bed pads for Clint Ober back in 2001 or so. And in the process I got grounded. I thought that grounding might be able to help my hands and my heart. I had had open-heart surgery the year before.

"The grounding helped indeed. My hands stopped hurting. I don't recall exactly how long it took, but I remember that I was significantly impressed to the point that I continued doing it. Even to this day, if I travel or otherwise go without sleeping grounded for two or three days, my hands will start hurting again, as well as the shoulders, neck, and other parts of my body where I have a touch of arthritis. As soon as I get home, I ground myself. Within one day, or even within hours, I can stop the pain. It disappears.

"I'm an avid golfer and have been so all my life. Now that I'm retired I play practically every day, and, even though I'm seventy-five, I'm still very competitive. In fact, I'm the champion at my club. I was a 2 to 3 handicap golfer in my younger days. Now I'm still at a 3 to 4 handicap level. None of my contemporaries are at my level anymore. All the guys I used to play with when I was younger and who played me even or beat me can't come close to me anymore. They have lost their capacity to play competitively. I have not. I play with the pros my age and I kick their tails. They can't believe it.

"I play golf grounded. I make a hole in the sole of my shoes and insert a conductive plug. I think that sleeping and playing grounded has something to do with being supple and able to take the physical beating caused by daily practice and playing. Most people my age stop being competitive because they can't take the abuse to their body. They can't practice, swing really hard, or push their games because it hurts. So they don't win. I can't beat the really good twenty- or thirty-year-old kids. Nothing hurts when they swing. But the older ones don't beat me."

EARTHING AND LAWN-BOWLING LONGEVITY

Shane Austin, Dumfries, Scotland, telecom engineer: "Since early 2012, my ninety-year-old grandfather Tommy Saville has been grounded daily and as a result went quickly from hurting and bad mobility to not hurting and good mobility.

"Tommy was a farmer and shepherd for sixty years and has kept active since retiring. He loves lawn bowling. While gardening one day, a heavy plank fell and crushed his foot. The foot became black and blue, and swollen. He kept bowling but his game was suffering, and he wasn't doing himself any good by not resting the foot.

"I heard about Earthing, and a couple of weeks after his accident I got an Earthing mat for him and me. After forty-eight hours, the swelling had decreased by a third, and after three weeks, it was about 80 percent reduced and he had regained full mobility! That's amazing when you consider his age. He was quickly back on his bowling game. Within two to three months, the rest of the swelling disappeared. His foot was back to 100 percent!

"I'd have bet a lot of money he wouldn't have made it through the 2012 bowling season if it weren't for Earthing powering him up. In 2013, he completed another successful bowling season.

"He uses his mat all the time. He carries it with him to bed and when he relaxes watching television.

"As for me and grounding, I severely twisted and sprained my ankle after a bad bike fall in 2012, and within three weeks it was healed. In four weeks I was back to running 10K! Amazing. The recommendation was six to eight weeks' rest."

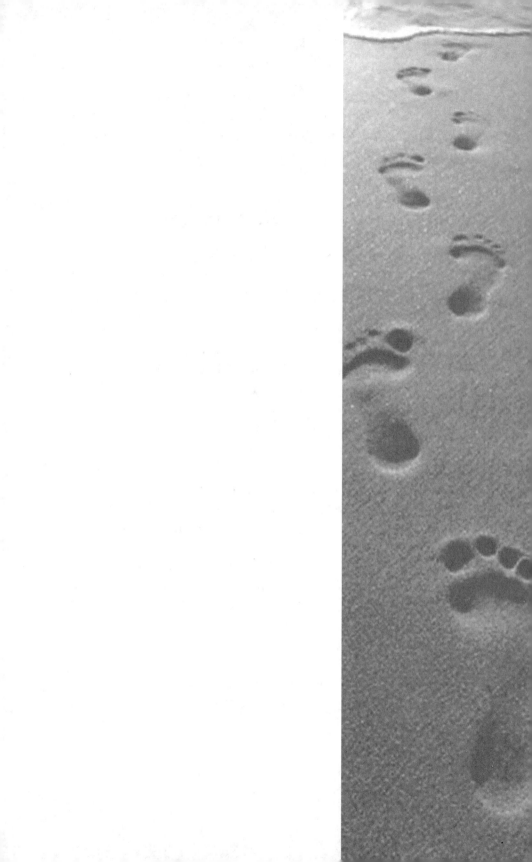

CHAPTER 15

The Animal Connection: Earthing and Pets

C lint Ober recalls an incident from his youth and growing up on a farm in Montana that left a vivid image in his memory: "One day while tending to some cattle with my dad we came upon a calf lying on the ground with a portion of its intestines hanging out of a large gash in its stomach. The mother cow was standing nearby as if protecting the calf. We were not sure what had happened. Maybe dogs or wolves attacked it, or it had gotten tangled up in some barbed wire. My dad took a needle and some coarse thread out of a saddlebag and went over and rolled the calf onto its side. He told me to sit on the calf to hold it still. My dad then pushed the exposed intestines back in the calf's belly and then proceeded to sew her up. No antiseptics. No antibiotics. Upon completion, my dad said she would either live or die and there was nothing more we could do. We were several miles away from the barn. The weather was very cold and it was snowing. There was no way we could have taken the calf back to the barn.

"I didn't think much more about this incident until a week or so later when I saw the same calf running around with the other calves like nothing had happened. Thereafter, I often wondered why outdoor animals seemed to heal up naturally and quickly from wounds as compared to humans, or even indoor pets, who seemed to take much longer to heal and to need excessive treatment and care. So many times I noticed sick animals lying in a dark corner on the Earth and then coming around seemingly healthy again.

"Whenever I asked veterinarians who treated both outdoor and indoor animals about this, they would just shrug and say the outdoor animals are out in Nature and that gives them something that indoor animals don't have. That something obviously includes more sunlight but, as I have learned, the natural healing energy of the Earth. They are connected."

ANIMALS NEED TO FEEL THE EARTH

Stephen R. Blake, D.V.M., San Diego, veterinarian: "As a holistic veterinarian with more than thirty years in practice, I have made it my goal to learn the natural ways animals keep themselves healthy by observation and study. The Earthing principle has been apparent to me since I was a child, growing up around animals. They like to dig in the ground, especially when they are stressed in any way.

"A very common example of an animal trying to ground himself is when they dig down into the carpeting or flooring of your home, when they are stressed or ill. They are trying to get to the concrete slab or get closer to the Earth. If you let them outside, they will do the same in the ground. Many times when a cat or dog is ill, you will find them outside under a bush where they have dug a hole to rest in. My feeling is they are tapping into the energy field of the Earth and benefiting from the infinite source of negative electrons and other intrinsic healing properties of the Earth.

"I have had cases where owners were reluctant to take their cats out into the yard because of fear of them running away and/or getting fleas. I would try and convince them to either use a harness and/or create a pen where the pet could walk on the Earth. When the owners did so, I usually found that animals improved both physically and behavior-wise.

"One cat named Charlie lived in a multi-cat family that was not allowed outside. Charlie was urinating in the home. I convinced the owner to start taking him outside for an hour a day. Immediately, the cat stopped his urinating behavior inside. His overall energy improved as well.

"I recall another cat named Minny. She had been an indoor cat for over a decade. She was irritable and did not like to be touched by anyone. Once her owners started taking her outside and letting her roam in the yard, her entire attitude changed. She was more social and affectionate.

"I have treated many animals who have spent their entire lives in a high-rise building without any contact with the Earth. I have advised their owners to ground their animals in some way. Preferably, take their animals outside as much as possible and let them have contact with the Earth's surface. Indoors, you can provide a grounding surface for an animal with a copper wire attached to a metallic water pipe or an Earthing product. I suggest placing it in their bed so they get maximum contact time with the Earth throughout the day and night.

"You would be surprised how just a simple thing like contact with the Earth can make a difference."

GROUNDED DOGS

Several years ago, pet health writer C.J. Puotinen and her husband obtained a grounding bed pad, which improved their sleep. "My husband was a professor of mechanical engineering," she says, "and the theory behind this simple technology made perfect sense to him." A writer of books and magazine articles about holistic pet care, Puotinen wondered whether bed pads could improve the life of animals as well. She contacted Dale Teplitz, a health and energy medicine researcher who had helped conduct several Earthing studies over the years. The two teamed up to design an experiment for dogs in 2007 utilizing a prototype grounded pad.

Together, they identified sixteen canines with histories of unresolved arthritic pain, fatigue, anxiety, hip dysplasia, chronic coughs, old injuries, and emotional problems. For the purpose of the study, the animals slept grounded on the pad for four to six weeks. The owners kept daily and weekly logs of their observations. During the experiment, the animals were only allowed to be naturally grounded for several minutes a day when relieving themselves outdoors.

The typical feedback from owners who kept detailed records included improvements in energy, stamina, flexibility, joint mobility, muscle tone, calmness, sleep, and signs of pain such as limping, stiffness, tentative movements, low activity levels, or a reluctance to jump, play, or move quickly, according to Teplitz.

"After the trial ended, some of the owners stopped using the pads briefly to see if there was any difference in the animals," she added. "They reported seeing pretrial signs starting to return. That really made them believe in grounding even more."

A Chipper Chip

One participant in the experiment was Chip McGrath, a retired racing Greyhound who belonged to Roberta Mikkelsen of Pearl River, New York. Chip had a bad limp because of joint stress and racing injuries, a result of hard running at speeds up to 45 miles per hour. The dog had also reinjured his leg and was unable to jump onto the couch or into the car for nearly a year.

"Now, thanks to the Earthing mat, he does both all the time," said Mikkelsen in 2009. "He has no evidence of pain or joint problems. He's more playful, jumps and runs more, tolerates longer walks, and has far more energy than before. He still limps a bit, but the veterinarian says that's because of the corns on his paws from his earlier racing days."

One of the surprising "side effects" of grounding was an "amazing mental change" in Chip within three weeks of sleeping grounded. "He had always been anxious and afraid of thunder, fireworks, and other loud noises," said Mikkelsen. "He would pant, pace, shake, and hide during storms until the storm was over. Greyhounds who have been raced a lot seem to develop lots of fears, and Chip sure had his share. But that behavior just stopped. The Earthing mat seems to have taken the fear out and calmed him. Now, when the weather is stormy, he is as calm as can be and goes readily off to sleep. For two years in a row now, he has even slept through Fourth of July fireworks."

Impressed by the improvements in her dog, Mikkelsen obtained an Earthing sheet for her husband who suffered with pain from spinal compression fractures. Her husband experienced minor relief, but Mikkelsen was totally surprised about what happened to her own pain problem.

"For two months, my fingers, elbows, hips, and knees had all been hurting, a consequence of overdoing it while laying a brick patio in my backyard," she recalled. "When I got up out of a chair, I could hardly walk. I had to wait a few moments before I could get moving. Within three days of Earthing, my pain disappeared and hasn't returned. I am as spry as before. This was totally unexpected."

Chip McGrath passed on in 2012, at the age of 13. Mikkelsen told us that "he would always snuggle up on his mat and seemed to be content and in less pain. When he slept, it was a deep peaceful sleep. After going out and returning to the house, he would head straight for his Earthing bed even though he had four other beds! I am now left with two senior whippets. They take turns Earthing and I believe that is one reason they are so calm and peaceful."

IMPROVED QUALITY—AND LENGTH—OF LIFE

Sandra Wong, Boulder, Colorado, violinist and music teacher: "Raffie is my eleven-year-old Great Pyrenees. He suffers from severe arthritis and multiple structural issues, including soft tissue laxity in both front legs. I felt I had exhausted all options for helping him with his extreme pain, including medication that made him sick to his stomach. I was approaching the difficult decision to put him down. Then a friend suggested grounding and I obtained an Earthing throw product for him. The results were striking. Within minutes, he appeared to relax significantly. Within several days I could see marked shifts in his movements, and in a week's time, much greater ease of motion compared to before.

"He either lies on top of it or I drape it over his whole body. He appears to deeply and completely relax. His breathing shifts to deep, slower breaths and his whole musculature relaxes. He will sleep soundly for hours at a time, compared to the short breaths he constantly took before, indicating pain. When he gets up, he acts deeply refreshed, moving with greater ease of motion, even rolling onto his back just for fun (something I hadn't seen for months). It was to the point that it would be midday before he would want to get up to go out and he would want to come right back in. He now wants to go out first thing in the morning and enjoys walking around the yard barking at squirrels. He is back to asking me to go out multiple times a day. I thought the days of him going bang, bang, bang on the back door were long gone! Now it's music to my ears again! He is still an elderly dog with serious physical challenges but the difference that Earthing has made to his quality of life is huge. He is enjoying life as a dog again without such intense pain. I know his time is limited but I am deeply grateful for the time and most important, the added quality of life.

"As a side note, I am a violinist and music teacher, and started using Earthing patches on my wrists, elbows, and left shoulder, where years of playing and repetitive use had created inflammation. My pain has significantly cleared up."

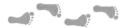

Shirley Evans, Calgary, Canada, retired teacher: "Abby the tabby was our rescue cat since she was a kitten. She lived her entire life, and until the end, a healthy life inside the house. Early in 2013, at age thirteen, she got acutely sick and for about two weeks stopped eating and drinking. She lost a lot of weight in the process.

"The veterinarian who saw her diagnosed severe pancreatitis, the worst case she had seen at the clinic. Abby spent two days there and received intravenous fluids. She was near death. The veterinarian said there was nothing to be done. She gave me painkillers, and said to try to make the cat as comfortable as I could until death came.

"I suddenly thought, why don't I ground her? I had nothing to lose. So I placed the Earthing mat at her favorite spot on the couch. She was so sick that she just stayed there, on the mat. At times, I also grounded myself on the couch and sat Abby on my lap so that she, too, would be grounded. She seemed to like being grounded. She looked comfortable.

"After one day of grounding she got up and, quite unsteady on her legs, walked to her water/food dish. She looked at it for a minute and then walked back to the sofa. She did this several times. Finally, as she wobbled back again to check out the dish, she drank and ate a little. Then at intervals, she kept going back—again and again—to eat and drink.

"Slowly, she regained her strength and kept showing signs of getting better, and returning to her sweet-natured little self. She even would also go out to sun herself on the concrete patio.

"Six months later she had an acute attack and didn't survive it. Earthing provided her an extra six months to live and she enjoyed the time. She thought going outside on the patio was really 'big time.'

"Earthing has also helped me with my atrial fibrillation and high blood pressure. I no longer take medications and I can only thank Earthing for it. The inner calmness seems to steady the heartbeat."

EARTHING AND SEIZURES

We have heard informally from a number of people that Earthing helps reduce the intensity and frequency of seizures in both adults and children.

Up to 5 percent of dogs suffer from seizures as well, and it is often an inherited condition; it is rarer in felines. The term epilepsy is used when seizures (also known as convulsions) recur. It is considered to be a brain disorder that results in a disturbance of normal electrochemical impulses of the nerve cells leading to strange sensations, emotions, seizures, muscle spasms, and even loss of consciousness.

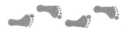

Cynthia Fertal, Bethlehem, Pennsylvania: "ChaCha, our fifteen-year-old long-haired Chihuahua, was experiencing lengthier and more frequent seizures as she got older. They would happen twice a month and then sometimes even weekly. It was heartbreaking to watch. She would lose complete control as her body would get stiff as a board, while her head was thrown back and her eyes wide open in terror. All we could do is hold her tight so she would not hurt herself in the process, until it was over.

"About nine plus months ago, my husband and I obtained an Earthing sheet. ChaCha sleeps in our bed as well and we observed, to our amazement, that the seizures immediately stopped the day we put the Earthing sheet on the bed. She has not even had a twitch or any of the gagging/coughing reactions on display when the seizures were in effect. Obviously, we have been thrilled to know that she no longer suffers with those debilitating seizures. The sheet has also helped with her arthritis and the awful effects of Lyme disease. She now runs around normally instead of limping. She is almost like a young puppy again. It's amazing!"

THE GROUNDED COCKATOO

Don Scott, an aviculturist in Escondido, California, founded the Chloe Sanctuary, a rescue shelter for cockatoos and parrots. He finds "foster" homes for the birds and trains people how to handle them as pets.

His experience with Chloe, the namesake of his sanctuary, suggests that the use of a grounded perch may help prevent or minimize the common psychoses—screaming, pacing, biting, and feather destructive behavior—of caged birds.

"Something substantial changed after I installed a grounded perch in Chloe's cage," he said. That was in mid-2008. Chloe was a twenty-five-year-old umbrella cockatoo at the time. She had been rescued from previous owners unable to give her proper care.

When Chloe came into Scott's care in 2003, she had an established problem of feather-destructive behavior due to being left alone for weekends at a time. According to veterinary records, Chloe had apparently been doing this since 2000. Social birds like these do not do well in situations of sustained separation from those they consider their flock. Cockatoos mate for life and always remain within screeching distance of their mate except when caring for their young. This devotion applies to their human "mates" as well.

"Chloe has become much calmer with the grounded perch," according to Scott. "She used to intensely pull out her feathers. It was bad. She doesn't do that anymore. She may tug at her feathers a little bit now and then, but only at the tips and not at the base as she used to do.

"Before, she would sit a good deal of the time in the cage and show little interest in her environment. Now she forages more for food and plays more with her toys. She is more active and playful."

The perch consists of an 18-inch stainless steel bathroom grab bar that Scott bought at Home Depot. He mounted it on a 1-by-3-inch piece of pine, attached a copper wire and connected it to the ground terminal in a wall outlet.

The grounded perch is not the highest perch in the cage. It's in the middle. Birds prefer a high perch at night out of an instinct for safety. The higher the perch the less chance of being attacked.

"But Chloe prefers this lower perch and uses it consistently at night," said Scott. "Instinctively, she picked up something that attracted her. What's fascinating is that once the grounded perch became disconnected and I wasn't aware of it, Chloe immediately sensed some difference and ignored the perch and went back to the perch at the higher level. I wondered why this was happening and then I discovered the disconnection. After reconnecting, Chloe went back to sitting on the middle perch again."

Scott said that Chloe was initially upset by the new perch but quickly felt very comfortable on it, and without screaming to be let out of the cage. Since installing the perch, she stopped walking a "figure eight" repeated pattern on the cage door, another sign of wanting to get out.

CHAPTER 16

The Long-Term Connection: The Importance of Staying Connected

There's a popular saying that if you don't use it, you lose it. That certainly holds true for Earthing.

Terry Pocklington, a Northern California businessman, contacted us in early 2012 to report a significant improvement in his circulation after six months of Earthing for about thirty to forty-five minutes daily. Two years before, he had been dealing with poor circulation, and stiffness and loss of feeling in his feet. He often experienced difficulty walking at times. Sometimes, he said, he had to force himself out of bed for his morning walk. He first went on an antioxidant supplement program, felt some improvement, and later started Earthing, with even more dramatic improvement. He was now seeing a healthy rosy coloration in his feet.

"When Earthing, the bottom of my feet and mostly the balls of my feet have a sensation of warmth as if something different is occurring. It's as if there is a current flowing," he said. "The feeling in my feet has definitely improved."

Then, for eight months, beginning in November 2012, Terry got out of the habit. He stopped Earthing. Despite an active routine of exercise, he began noticing his energy lagging. When Earthing, he had been jogging up to two miles a day five to six times a week. On some days he could now only walk.

Then he remembered Earthing. Soon, he was able to get back to jogging with renewed energy. The feeling of warmth in his soles also returned.

In July 2013, he told us that Earthing created "positive results to my health, followed by negative results because of discontinuation, and then positive results again when I resumed. I now know that Earthing needs to be part of my daily wellness practice."

In 2011, we heard from Clover Calvet, a retired businesswoman and teacher in Fairfield, Iowa. She had been Earthing for a couple of years and having consistently deeper and more restful sleep, more energy, and a dramatic reduction in gum inflammation. "For two weeks after the departure of a house guest, I was suddenly feeling miserable with a lot of fatigue," she said. "My gums became sore again and I didn't sleep well at all. At first I thought it was a result of too much activity while playing host to my guest, but I finally discovered I had forgotten to plug in my Earthing sheet. Now all is well again. Sleep, energy, and gums good!"

Fabio Luiz Vieira, M.D., a Brazilian general practitioner, told us in 2012 that he had been sleeping better and feeling more energy. On a brief trip to Rio de Janeiro, he took his sheet with him. "The first night I had a very good night of sleep but the second one was terrible, superficial, and filled with nightmares," he said. "I was puzzled because until then I had been sleeping very well when grounded. In the morning when I was packing to return home, I discovered that the chambermaid had disconnected the sheet wire after the first night!"

Anita Moran, of Biddleford, Maine, reported in 2011 that since sleeping grounding she had major relief from arthritic pain in her right foot, something she had unsuccessfully tried to resolve for more than a decade. Two years later, she said the pain has not gone away completely, but what she has noticed is that "if I don't ground myself, it's worse. I went away for a weekend once and forgot the mat. My foot became more painful and inflamed and it took a few nights to get back to where I was."

One more thing. If you have pets, be aware of their potential for Earthing cord destruction. The following note from an Earthing enthusiast in Pittsburgh is a reminder: "I started sleeping on an Earthing sheet and became hooked on the good sleep. After some time, though, I began to feel lousy and again found I had a hard time falling asleep. I checked the sheet connection, and found that my son's cat had chewed it apart. After getting a replacement, I am once again sleeping like a baby."

Bottom line: Whether you connect to the Earth inside or outside,

MAKE SURE YOU STAY CONNECTED!

CHAPTER 17

The Future Connection: The Earthing Revolution Ahead

This book is a statement about Nature and health. Health is natural, and part of being naturally healthy and functioning optimally appears to involve connectedness to the Earth. Being disconnected seems to be both unnatural and unhealthy. The disconnect creates unnecessary suffering in the form of sickness, inflammation, pain, and poor sleep—the consequences of an electron deficiency. Connecting to the Earth remedies that deficiency and its consequences.

We think this book offers a relevant piece of the answer to T. H. Huxley's prodigious question about determining our place in Nature and our relationship to the cosmos. We live on our planet. But we have insulated ourselves from it—and at great cost. As a society, we are hurting and unhealthy, and we have been that way for quite a while. The health statistics indicate that we are no longer the hardy, red-blooded folks we used to be. We stress our bodies to the breaking point. We eat the wrong foods and don't exercise.

Back fifty years ago or so, with the emergence of medical insurance plans, people expected they'd be taken care of when they got old and there would be a pill for every illness. Today, there is a pill for practically every illness, but the pills don't particularly cure anything or make us healthier.

The late John Knowles, M.D., head of the Massachusetts General Hospital and the Rockefeller Foundation during the 1960s and 1970s, put it this way years ago: "People have been led to believe that national health insurance, more doctors, and greater use of high-cost, hospital-based technologies will improve health. Unfortunately, none of them will."

At the time, politicians and doctors had become increasingly concerned about the rising costs of health care. Sound familiar? Such costs were eating up about 8 percent of the domestic national product back then. Today, the percentage has more than doubled and is supposed to reach 20 percent in a few years! Politicians and doctors are still concerned, but concern hasn't helped much.

And the future?

Ouch! It hurts to look ahead.

HEALTH CARE CHANGE . . . FROM THE GROUND UP

According to a 2002 report from the United Nation's Department of Economic and Social Affairs, the global population is aging at a speed "without parallel in human history." Between 2000 and 2050, the proportion of people over sixty will double from 11 to 22 percent.

Aging populations represent serious economic, political, and social challenges for governments dealing with healthcare obligations. In the United States, as an example, aging baby boomers, 80 million strong, have started to reach sixty-five and are eligibile for Medicare's government-funded health insurance. This means a huge influx of people and age-related chronic health issues draining an already strained medical system. As a 2013 report in the *Journal of the American Medical Association* put it, there is an overall volume increase of years living with disability and illness because "individuals are living longer but are not necessarily in good health." Without any significant changes, the surge may break the Medicare coffers—and predictions for that have already surfaced.

The Council of State Governments, a leading multi-branch organization forecasting policy trends, said in a 2006 alert on chronic disease that along with more forecasted disease among the older population, there is also the issue of more children entering their teen years, college, and adulthood with diabetes, high blood pressure, and other effects of overweight, physical inactivity, and unhealthful eating. "Some experts estimate that the generation growing up today will be the first to live a shorter life than their parents and grandparents. This will have a tremendous effect on public resources and the ability of public agencies to provide healthcare and social services, while draining a critical U.S. resource—the workforce."

The status quo isn't working. The situation threatens the health of individuals, the family, and nations everywhere. Declining health is hardly an American monopoly. The health of all humanity is in crisis. The many ailments besetting the United States are symptomatic of a planetary catastrophe in the making before our eyes and headlined in the news every single day.

The analogy of raising cows may be appropriate here. If humans were cows, they would have to be taken out and shot. Who could afford the veterinary bill?

Health care, as it operates today, is impotent, exorbitant, and ineffective. Chronic disorders are out of control, and the solution is really not in the hands of government or insurers. It is in our hands. Our health, or lack of it, is by and large the result of how we live.

"Self-care is the only effective way to ensure good health and a longer, fuller life," wrote Joseph D. Beasley, M.D., and Jerry J. Swift, M.A., in an epic 1989 Ford Foundation book, *The Kellogg Report: The Impact of Nutrition, Environment & Lifestyle on the Health of Americans* (Bard College). "While there is a crying need for reforms of the healthcare system, the most needed reform of all is in our own attitudes—we patients must become activists for our own health."

These and many other similar admonitions have largely remained beyond the hearing range of most people, who persist in overeating unnatural food and avoiding physical activity. So we just become sicker and sicker.

Instead of focusing on health insurance, we need to emphasize health assurance. We reach that greater level of protection by removing the major sources of stress and toxicity in our lives. In this book, we propose one surprisingly and utterly simple means of helping to reach that goal.

EARTHING'S PARADIGM-CHANGING HEALTH AND ECONOMIC POTENTIAL

Earthing represents a discovery of the first magnitude, as potentially significant and globally sweeping as electricity, telephones, radio, television, and computers. Consider the changes that new technologies like these brought to society in their time. We are still riding the waves of innovation they generated in terms of jobs and economies. Earthing, like these concepts, is disruptive in that it changes how people live.

We believe that Earthing can change the way medicine itself is practiced, adding major effectiveness in healing while lowering the cost of treatments for many diseases. Keep in mind that the physiology of the grounded person appears to be different—in a more efficient and healthier way—than that of an ungrounded person.

As more research rolls out, we envision Earthing units being installed in spas and the clinics of health practitioners. We envision patients being grounded in hospitals and nursing homes. Sophisticated electrically operated equipment and instrumentation are grounded in medical and health-care facilities. The beds are grounded. Why not the patients in those beds?

Looking ahead, we believe that Earthing can generate a broad societal and economic overhaul.

Economies are based on businesses that create profits, jobs, and wealth. We think that Earthing offers a huge bonanza for business the world over. Earthing has the potential to benefit—and change—the world in many ways. It is equally available to the richest and the poorest, to both the industrialized and the developing world.

Earthing will affect all society—literally from the ground up, starting with the shoe industry. The simple insertion of a few cents of conductive carbon or some other similar material in the soles of shoes can bring people into contact again with the Earth's healing energy. The shoe manufacturing industry hasn't acted in bad faith, but its innovations have contributed to the rise of chronic illness. Here's a golden opportunity for the shoe industry to redeem and reinvent itself in the name of health . . . and expanded sales. What a glorious prospect! Every year a person buys at least one new pair of shoes. For a small investment on the part of the industry, so much good can be done in the marketplace. As a consumer, start asking about grounded shoes the next time you make a purchase. Create the demand!

Earthing has the potential to thoroughly revolutionize the bedding and mattress industry. Every eight years on average, people replace their mattresses in the United States. About 30 million are sold each year. And there is a mattress store for every 20,000 homes in America. Here is an industry that sells bed comfort in all forms: water, air, springs, foam, latex. But just by adding a few dollars' worth of conductive material to the mattress and connecting it to the Earth, it can improve the health of a society full of insomniacs. The new mattress bottom line will be: more comfort, better sleep, less pain, better health.

Imagine the rush to buy grounded mattresses!

Hotels have been spending billions on twenty-first century upgrades such as flat-screen TVs, wireless Internet, trendier bars, and fancier showers. Imagine the appeal of hotels offering weary travelers grounded mattresses to promote sleep and elimination of jet lag.

The shoe and mattress industry have blockbuster products to sell and, while they are at it, become a part of the healthcare industry. These are the best place to start the Earthing revolution. Is there any simpler kind of health reform than that? When you go out to purchase shoes and mattresses, you will simultaneously be buying better health for yourself.

There are innumerable business opportunities to bring the Earth's healing electrons up into our lives so that everyone lives grounded most of each and every day. Homes, offices, and schools need to be grounded. That includes floors, carpets, and furniture. Even cars can get a modified dose of grounding with a simple seat pad. All these basic parts of society's infrastructure can be inexpensively outfitted with conductive material, creating a whole Earthing industry to ground new and existing houses. Out of this will come whole new manufacturing, marketing, distributing, and installation industries, just like exists today with telephone or cable systems.

Think of how all this will impact the way we design our living and working environments. Can you imagine what effect all this will have on the health statistics we cited above? And on the economy of the world in terms of new jobs, careers, research, products, education, services, and even tax revenue for cash-strapped governments? For corporations, just think of what this will do to their own health insurance premiums and cost of doing business. Instead of a malignant cycle of bad health, we can create a benign cycle of good health that embraces and benefits both employers and employees alike.

Earthing is the future. Humanity needs to reconnect to the planet, to our natural electrical state, and to our natural state of good health.

It's so simple to do.

Our book is a bugle call. Wake up, people. Go out. Ground yourself. Reintroduce your bare feet to the ground. Sleep grounded, and, if you can, work grounded, play grounded, and watch TV grounded.

If you haven't done it by now, go sit or stand barefoot outside (weather permitting) for a half hour or so. If you have pain, see what difference it makes. Then ask yourself if reconnecting with the Earth might be the most amazing health discovery *you* have ever made.

We think that reconnecting with the Earth is amazing and may, in fact, be *the* most important health discovery ever.

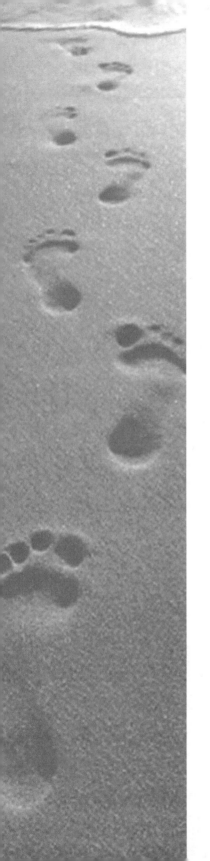

Appendices

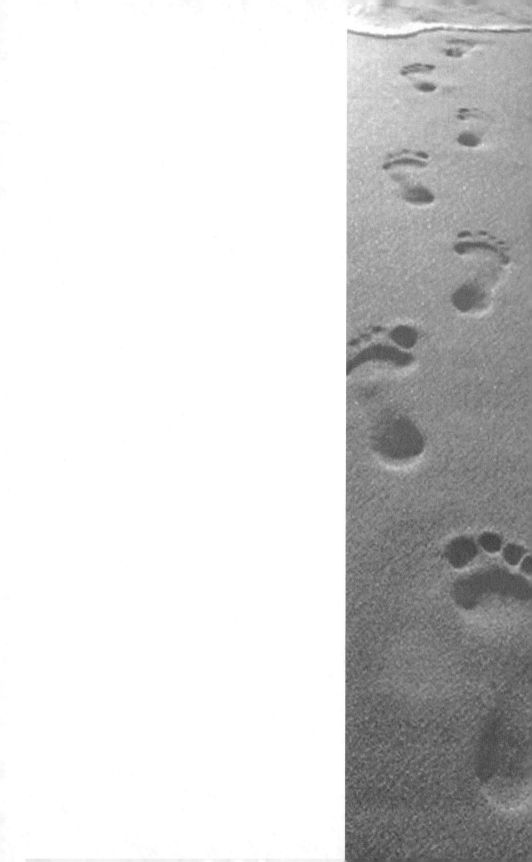

APPENDIX A

The Physics of Earthing— Simplified

By Gaétan Chevalier, Ph.D.
Visiting Scientist, Developmental and Cell Biology Department,
University of California at Irvine

After twenty years of research in electrophysiology and biofeedback, and another ten with Earthing, I have come to regard the contemporary biochemical model of the human body as severely lacking. What's largely missing is a fundamental understanding of the bioelectrical nature of our physiology.

The body is a highly intelligent electrobiochemical system that is strongly influenced by its internal electrical environment. Countless electrical charges within this system regulate countless biochemical reactions, including enzymatic transformations, protein formation, and pH (acid/alkaline) balance. In this complex arrangement, the Earth's surface electric potential serves as the body's stabilizing reference point or ground. As I have learned through my research and that of my colleagues, contact with the surface of the Earth maintains the body's electrical stability and the normal functioning of its self-regulating and self-healing mechanisms. The ground thus acts as the very same stabilizing resource for both the body and electrical systems throughout the world.

Our research leads us to conclude that a lack of grounding leads to internal electrical instability that in turn results in physiological dysfunction. Think of multiple domino effects happening simultaneously. They lead to precursors or aggravating factors for numerous disorders. In previous times, before our modern lifestyle separated us from the Earth's ground reference, the body typically had its natural hookup to electrical stability. In one way or another, such as by being barefoot or using animal hides for bedding and footwear that permitted conductivity, humans had ordinary and routine conductive contact with the Earth.

Let's explore the details of this electrical connection.

THE EARTH'S NEGATIVE CHARGE

The surface of the Earth is the most negatively charged entity in the immediate human environment. But as we lift off the surface of the planet and gain altitude, the electric potential (meaning, the level of electrical energy or the potency of the electric charge) increases 100 to 200 volts with every meter (about 3 feet), depending on location. This is a well-established scientific fact.

Why, you might be thinking, wouldn't one get electrocuted from all that voltage in the air? You don't because the air close to the surface of the Earth has insulating qualities, rendering the electric current near the ground very low, close to zero. Simply put, without current you can't be zapped.

Let's now climb higher into the sky, up into the wild blue yonder. At several kilometers (miles) of altitude, the increase of atmospheric voltage begins to slow. At around 100 kilometers (62.5 miles), the increase stops. That's because the atmosphere becomes a conductor. At this height, the sun's rays are powerful enough to take electrons away from air molecules (even to break up molecules) and, in so doing, generate ions (charged particles). Thus, scientists gave the name "ionosphere" to this region of the atmosphere.

In fair weather, when the sky is blue with few to no clouds, the difference in electric potential is 250,000 to 500,000 volts between the Earth's surface and the ionosphere. Visualize this system as two conductors, one at zero volts (the ground) and the other at 250,000 to 500,000 volts at an altitude of about 100 kilometers.

As mentioned, fair weather atmosphere below the ionosphere is not a good conductor, especially close to the ground. But it is not really a perfect insulating medium either. A very small current of electrons escapes from the ground at a rate of approximately 1 milliamp (mA) per square kilometer (equivalent to a power loss of 1 microwatt per square meter). This phenomenon is known as the "fair weather current" and is a component of an immense natural activity called the "global electrical circuit" (see Figure A-1).

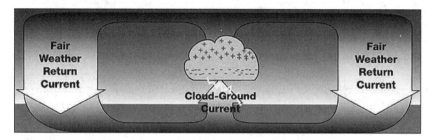

Figure A-1. Global electrical circuit. A current coming up from the ground at the location of lightning (depositing electrons into the earth) and returning to the ground elsewhere. *Source:* NASA/MSFC (Dooling)

The global circuit is primarily recharged by cumulonimbus (storm) clouds. During an active thunderstorm, the collection of clouds generates an average current of about 1 amp down to the surface of the Earth. There are an estimated 1,000 to 2,000 thunderstorms happening globally at any one time, and collectively these storms produce as many as 5,000 lightning strikes per minute. Thus, an electrical current of 1,000 to 2,000 amps is continually transferring a negative charge to the surface of the Earth and an equal and opposite charge to the upper atmosphere. More recent research has shown that heavy rains also contribute to the negative charge of the Earth's surface.

To simplify a very complex phenomenon, it is understood by scientists that activity within the storm clouds produces a buildup of negative charges at the bottom of the clouds, while the top of the clouds become positively charged, as depicted in Figure A-1. Simultaneously, positive charges build up in the ground below the clouds. At some point, the buildup above and below becomes so great that lightning results. It is a matter of opposite charges attracting. Lightning involves a transfer of a massive amount of negative charges to the ground.

WHAT HAPPENS TO THE NEGATIVE CHARGE
IN THE GROUND?

In the ground, particularly close to the surface, the overall negative charge creates the Earth's electric field. This charge takes the shape of a virtually limitless and continuously renewed reservoir of free electrons. This unseen sea of electrons is subject to a wide array of rhythms and movements according to stimuli from the sun and moon, and from processes going on in the atmosphere and inside the Earth itself.

Here are several examples of electron movements:

- **Circadian rhythms.** During the day the sun gives much energy to the electrons on the surface of the Earth, making them vibrate faster; at night this energy dissipates, making the electrons vibrate slower.

- **Telluric currents.** Electrons in the ground are maximally energized by midday solar rays. This effect generates huge electric currents that sweep electrons from the geographical zone of highest solar intensity to adjacent zones of lesser intensity. These movements, referred to as "telluric currents," accompany the sun's overhead position in a twenty-four-hour cycle. Together with the local electron vibrations, they serve to synchronize the body's internal biological clocks and rhythms with the immediate geoelectrical environment.

- **Schumann resonance.** An example of a faster electron vibration is the so-called Schumann resonance, a natural and omnipresent electromagnetic signal generated by lightning. With a primary frequency of 7.8 Hz, this frequency falls in the alpha frequency band of brain waves that corresponds to a calm, meditative state.

These are not the only types of energies and energy fields existing on, near, and under the surface of the Earth. Another is the familiar geomagnetic field used to determine north with a compass. It is also a source of stabilizing and synchronizing frequencies but the electrons in the Earth are probably more important for us in that respect. It must be so, otherwise jet lag would not exist. When a person exits a plane after traveling through multiple time zones, the local geomagnetic field frequencies do not resynchronize the person's circadian rhythm and eliminate or reduce jet lag. Such modulation requires physical contact with the Earth—that's Earthing. This fact strongly suggests that the circadian rhythm and telluric currents of the Earth's electrons represent a more powerful source of stabilizing and synchronizing frequencies than the geomagnetic field.

Other types of energies and energy fields include heat (an emission of electromagnetic fields in the infrared band) and radioactive emissions from radioisotopes such as radium and radon produced by the decay of uranium and thorium below the ground.

THE DIFFERENCE BETWEEN THE EARTH'S ENERGY AND STANDARD ELECTRICITY

The Earth's electric field is mainly a continuous direct current (DC)–producing field. Throughout history, life on the planet has attuned our biology to this subtle field. By comparison, home-wiring systems in the United States use a 60 cycle per second alternating current (AC), and, in other parts of the world, a 50 cycle per second current is common. Unless at very low frequency (less than 40 cycles per second) and/or low power, alternating current is foreign to our biology. AC and other forms of man-made environmental electromagnetic fields are being researched as possible factors in a variety of stress-related responses and ailments.

WHAT HAPPENS ELECTRICALLY INSIDE YOUR BODY WHEN YOU ARE GROUNDED?

Scientists have made the arbitrary agreement—accepted globally—that the level of electric energy on the Earth's surface corresponds to an electric potential of zero. It does not mean the Earth is bereft of energy. If that were the case, there could be no electrons in the ground. Rather, this is a measurement standard that assigns everything above the surface of the Earth an electric potential higher than zero.

When you make bare-skin contact with the Earth, almost instantly, and practically at the speed of light, the electric potential of the body equalizes with the potential of the Earth. The initial flow of electrons and energy between the Earth and your body establishes an electric path. At any given time, this flow of electrons is very small but very significant.

Roger Applewhite, an electrical engineer, showed in an experiment that grounding decreases the 60-Hz-induced body voltage in a typical room by a factor of about 70, bringing it to an extremely minimal background level (electrical "noise") present in the environment. In addition, Polish researchers Karol and Pawel Sokal have measured how movement (standing up and lying down) affects the electrical potentials and currents on the surface and interior of the body. In their experiment, they found significant fluctuations when someone is not grounded—changes that were prevented with grounding. Their findings show that Earthing creates a stable electrical environment for the body by preventing external 50-Hz electromagnetic fields or internal currents from interfering with natural bioelectrical functions. (See Appendix G for more details on these studies.)

HOW ELECTRONS MOVE THROUGH YOUR BODY

Unlike electrical wiring, which uses copper to conduct electricity, the human body obviously conducts its electrical business without such wires to carry electrons. Those of us involved in Earthing research have some theories about how electrons gain access and are transported through the body even faster than in copper wiring. Some of these include:

- **The meridian system.** A series of interconnecting pathways within the body through which energy is thought to flow. Each pathway, or meridian, is linked to a specific organ. If you have your feet on the ground, this explanation would suggest that electrons enter via the K1-acupuncture point on the bottom of the foot and are distributed from the kidney meridian to other meridians, and then to the entire body.

- **The sweat glands.** Another access point may be through the sweat glands, which are found in high concentration on the bottoms of the feet, the palms of the hands, and the forehead. Each sweat gland receives several nerve fibers that branch out into bands of one or more axons and encircle the individual tubules of the secretory gland. Capillaries are also interwoven among sweat tubules.

- **The bloodstream.** This possibility is suggested by research showing that the electric potential in veins equalizes almost immediately with that of the Earth when someone is grounded. More evidence comes from the increase of red blood cell zeta potential (the negative charge on the surface of a red blood cell).

- **The living matrix.** A conductive network of connective tissue and filaments inside and outside cells that provides systemic informational and energetic connections throughout the body; this system may also provide storage space for "extra" electrons.

- **The autonomic nervous system (ANS).** This is the part of the nervous system that regulates functions like heart and respiration rates, digestion, perspiration, urination, and even sexual arousal, and that has branches everywhere in the body. The most likely ANS elements for electron transit are free nerve endings. These nonspecialized structures terminate within the epidermis, in hair follicle receptors (unencapsulated nerve endings wrapped around hair follicles), and in branches of peripheral nerves in the dermis. The latter includes smaller offshoots toward the surface (often near sweat glands or hair follicles) and larger ones in deeper layers (often running parallel to blood vessels). It is also possible that electrons "hop on" nerves and then end up in the bloodstream, where they are transported through the body by uric acid or other antioxidants present in the blood. If electrons can be transported with nerve impulses directly from the ANS to the central nervous system, they could be redirected anywhere at the speed of nerve impulses (10–100 meters per second).

Electrons are extremely reactive and it is very unlikely that they move by themselves without becoming attached to different molecules. More research is clearly needed to determine the pathways and transformations involving electrons.

HOW FAST DO ELECTRONS FLOW INTO THE BODY?

Electrons move very slowly even in a copper wire. When they enter the body through the feet, they immediately migrate upward. This flow of electrons might take twenty to thirty minutes to reach your belly.

Our research shows that some kind of healing starts to happen about twenty to thirty minutes after grounding the feet. For example, you might sense less pain first in the knees, followed by some relief in the back, and then the neck. Where you first experience relief depends on where you have made contact with the Earth on your body. It would take less time though if you put an Earthing patch or a grounding mat right near or on the source of some local pain. There is simply less distance for the electrons to travel to have an effect. That's what we often recommend to people seeking rapid relief from local pain or injury.

Let's examine the issue of electron speed in more technical detail, using the example of a 9-volt battery. Take a copper wire, fit a resistor onto it, and connect the ends to the positive and negative terminals of the battery. The current starts flowing from the positive terminal of the battery to the negative terminal. Positive charges are what make the copper material itself and so they cannot move. But the electrons move. They leave the negative terminal and flow to the positive terminal through the wire. Their motion is regulated by the resistor. Without it, all the electrons in the battery would travel to the positive terminal at the same time, melting the copper wire in the process. If you touched the wire, you would get burned.

Because a current is defined by the movement of positive charges, many people think that positive charges flow from the positive terminal to the negative terminal. However, it is the movement of the electrons from the *negative* terminal to the *positive* terminal that produces the current. The misconception dates back to dear old Benjamin Franklin who, through his experiments with kites and not knowing the exact nature of electricity, thought that a positively charged electric "fluid" was flowing into the wire.

We know now that electrons are always the flowing entities when there is a current in a conducting wire. The velocity of electrons moving into the wire (technically called the "drift velocity") is very slow. For a copper wire 1 millimeter (mm) in diameter carrying a steady current of 3 amps, the drift velocity is only about 0.24 mm per second—a quarter of a millimeter per second (about 1/100th of an inch per second)! And yet, the current flows extremely fast.

To explain how a slow electron flow can produce a very fast current, I'll use the example of a grounded person. In this scenario, the human body plays the role of both the copper wire and the resistor. (This is because the body is not as good a conductor as copper; it offers some resistance to the current of electrons from the ground.) The negative terminal is the Earth. The positive terminal is represented by the positively charged particles (positive ions) in the air. The protective effect against the positive ions in the air offered by the Earth connection is established almost at the speed of light, 186,000 miles per second. This means that the electric current flowing through the body neutralizes the positive ions coming in contact with the body almost instantaneously. Knowing that even in such an excellent conductor as copper electrons move very slowly, how can this be? An analogy may help our understanding.

In Figure A-2 below, a narrow tube or straw is filled with beads. The diameter of the tube accommodates the beads only in a line. If you push the bead on the left side into the full tube, a bead pops out the other side almost instantaneously. The entering bead on the left has moved only the distance of its diameter. It is now the last bead inside the tube on the left side and yet the *current* of beads has moved very fast. The last bead on the right side was pushed out almost instantaneously. Each bead inside

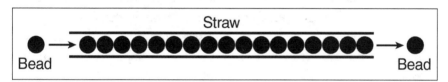

Figure A-2. The "straw-bead" effect. A bead introduced into the left end of the straw moves very little yet the bead at the far right end pops out almost instantly.

the tube moved a distance of one-bead diameter only and yet the *current* of beads (the propagation of the small movements of each bead) has moved through the tube almost instantaneously. All the beads inside the tube moved forward almost simultaneously. In principle, there is no limit to the length of the tube; the current can flow this way even if the tube is many miles long. This is also true if the tube is in a vertical position. This is because electrons, which are like the beads in the figure, have such a small mass that their electric field, which is much stronger than gravity, pushes them up easily against gravity, even if the tube is many miles (kilometers) long.

The "straw-bead" analogy helps us begin to understand how electrons move in a conductor. Electrons repel each other because they have the same negative electric charge. (Remember, same electric charges repel each other; opposite electric charges attract each other.) Because of this repelling effect between electrons, when an electron moves forward, it pushes forward all electrons ahead of it—just like the left bead pushed forward all the beads in the tube. This is what happens in a wire connected to both terminals of a battery. The slow movement of electrons in a wire also happens in the body and yet, at the same time, their slow movement collectively produces a fast current because of the "straw-bead" effect. The body is protected almost instantaneously by Earthing because the fast current cancels out the effects of low-frequency electromagnetic fields and/or the positive particles in the air very quickly.

The slow drift velocity of electrons helps explain a number of observations in regard to Earthing:

1. It takes about twenty to thirty minutes for the healing response to start once a person is grounded.

2. When people stand or sit on the Earth, or are grounded via electrode patches placed on the soles of their feet, they often start feeling tingling and warmth rise in their body. The sensation starts in the feet, then progresses to the shins and calves, and after about twenty minutes reaches the trunk and, finally, the head.

3. Grounding speeds wound healing. Wounds heal faster than normal (ungrounded). They heal even faster if an Earthing patch is placed close to the location of the wound.

4. Grounding reduces inflammation. Inflammation of the elbow, for example, will clear with the feet touching the ground. However, the inflammatory condition will be dissipated much faster if grounded electrode patches are placed on or near the elbow.

A NEW HEALTH AND HEALING FRONTIER

As a researcher involved primarily with the physics of bioelectricity and how the body produces and uses electrical energy, I find it amazing that at this point in the human time line—the beginning of the twenty-first century—we are just starting to scientifically explore the dynamics and benefits to health that come from direct contact with the electric planet we live on. The studies I have been involved with have yielded a fascinating picture of what happens when we connect to the Earth. To me, it's as if a switch is somehow turned on and the body's inner workings start functioning more vitally and robustly.

To be sure, our studies are few in number, but they strongly suggest a powerful, positive, and rapid shift in the physiology that may one day give rise to whole new definitions of what is normal. We have so much more to learn from the exploration of what truly appears to be a vast and magnificent health and healing frontier for humans everywhere on the planet.

For additional information regarding the science of grounding, please visit the Earthing Institute website at www.earthinginstitute.net.

Technical Notes on Grounding and Earthing Methods

Physicists and electrical engineers have chosen the Earth as the most obvious "ground," or reference point, for all electrical power grids. The Earth provides a reference voltage, that is, the ground or zero potential against which all other voltages are established and measured. There is no absolute electric potential. What is measured is the difference in electric potential between two points—one being the Earth, the reference point.

What Exactly Is a Ground?

A ground is defined as a conductive object that makes a direct electrical connection to Earth and has the ability to absorb or dissipate an electrical charge, thereby maintaining a grounded object at the stable electrical potential of the Earth. Grounding is central to the safe and stable usage of electricity. A ground connection serves as an electrical "sink" that minimizes the susceptibility of electromagnetic interference in communication systems; reduces the risk of equipment damage due to lightning; eliminates electrostatic buildup, which can damage system components; and helps protect people who service and repair electrical, electronic, and computer equipment.

In effect, an electrical ground drains away any unwanted buildup of electrical charge. When a device or person is connected to an Earth ground, that device or person will equalize with, and maintain, the stable electrical potential of the Earth.

An "Earth ground" usually consists of a ground rod driven into the Earth.

Earthing Methods and Considerations

We expect that after reading this book many people will want to experiment with Earthing in order to experience the effects that Earthing may have on their health and sleep.

The easiest method, of course, is as simple as routinely going outdoors and placing your bare feet directly on the Earth for thirty minutes at a time. But being barefoot is not always an option.

We have described a variety of personal Earthing products in the book that we call "barefoot substitutes." They include conductive floor and desk mats, sheets, bands, and patches that are intended for indoor use. They are connected to the Earth via a special cord. One end of the cord snaps on to the product and the other end can be attached to a ground rod or plugged into the ground port of a grounded wall outlet. Many of these items are now commercially available.

These systems were originally developed for use in proof-of-concept Earthing studies. Ways were needed to Earth people for study purposes when they were confined to one place during a testing period. From the start, many study participants and researchers requested Earthing systems for themselves, friends, and families, leading to further development and testing of various Earthing applications for indoor home use. Some proved to be functional and effective. Others, less so.

The primary concern in developing these home/office applications was to ensure both effectiveness and safety. In this process, the following facts became clear:

1. The most effective Earthing system in the studies consisted of a ground rod placed directly in the Earth with a ground wire running into the home and connected directly to the Earthing sheet, mat, etc. Still, most people who plug into a properly grounded wall outlet in their home or office report similar health benefits as those using dedicated ground rods. For best results, test the outlet first with a simple outlet checker for proper grounding or have an electrician check your electrical ground system.

2. Many individuals have experimented with common personal electro-static discharge (ESD) grounding systems for Earthing that are used in the electronics industry. They are designed to prevent the buildup of static electricity on the body, which could otherwise damage the microchips and hardware that employees handle when building or repairing computers and electronic equipment. Such ESD grounding devices are generally connected to the third-prong ground port of an electrical outlet. In factories where employees use EDS grounding systems, an electrical engineer or electrician will test and verify that the electrical ground is in good working order before allowing employees to connect themselves to this system.

ESD systems slowly dissipate static electricity on workers. By comparison, Earthing systems are conductive, meaning they instantly equalize the body with, and maintain the body at, Earth potential and are meant to simulate the natural, timeless human experience of being barefoot on the Earth outside. Earthing research has demonstrated that holding the body at Earth potential (simulating being barefoot outside) produces significant results on measurements related to inflammation, blood electrodynamics, and autonomic nervous system function.

There is no scientific evidence we are aware of relating to the effect of ESD systems on physiology, and thus have no way to objectively compare ESD to Earthing. ESD products are meant for industrial use. The Earthing design has been shown in repeated experiments, published in a variety of journals, to generate distinct changes in physiology and for which ESD products, meant for industrial use to prevent common static from damaging electronic components, have not been documented to do.

We have informally tested ESD products and found that they do not generate the same electrophysiological changes as does Earthing. While ESD products may produce some benefits, people have told us that ESD products do not produce the same experience and results as Earthing.

All ESD ground cords contain a 1-megohm resistor. A 1-megohm resistor allows 60 Hz EMF-induced body voltage to drop by 90 percent. Earthing products have a built-in 100k-ohm resistor in all ground cords for safety and allow 60 Hz EMF-induced body voltage to drop by 99 percent. Earthing's ability to bring and hold the body at Earth's potential restores the body's natural electrical state and facilitates inflammation reduction.

3. Many individuals who live in apartments and high-rise buildings ask if they can use the electrical ground system in their building for Earthing. From our experience, the electrical ground system in a building —that is, the use of wall outlets— is the only option that most people living in multi-story buildings will have unless they can drop a long wire out the window and connect it to a ground rod in the soil below.

   In general, a house or building electrical ground system will work for Earthing, as all electrical ground systems are connected directly to a ground rod driven into the Earth. However, there are certain problems that may be encountered:

   • Most residential homes built in the United States before the 1960s do not have an electrical ground system. Many of these homes have been remodeled with the old-style outlets being replaced with newer fixtures containing a ground port. In appearance, it may look as if the home has an electrical ground system, but there may not be an actual ground wire installed and connected to the newer ground port outlets. Thus, in many older homes there is no ground system. In these cases, use of a dedicated Earth ground rod system is the only option.

   • Some home electrical outlets are miswired. The most common wiring error is that of the ground and neutral being reversed. In order to verify that electrical ground outlets are correctly wired, inexpensive outlet-wiring checkers are available at all hardware and electrical retail outlets. Always check the outlet before using an Earthing product.

Lightning

One of the most common technical questions asked about Earthing is: Do I have to worry about lightning if I am grounded to the Earth?

Lightning is a massive natural phenomenon that is unpredictable and challenging to totally protect against. It is poorly understood. The following will help you understand how and usually when lightning occurs and what is your likelihood of being hit when grounded to the Earth.

Most lightning strikes occur in the summer during the afternoon (70 percent between noon and 6:00 PM). As the air temperature warms, evaporation increases. The warm moist air rises and forms fluffy cumulus clouds. As the moisture accumulates, the clouds darken and change into cumulonimbus or thunderstorm clouds with a flattened base and puffy top reaching as high as 40,000 feet. The upper portion of a thunderstorm cloud develops a positive electrical charge, and the bottom of the cloud develops a negative charge. Negative charges repel negative charges and attract positive charges. So, as the thundercloud passes overhead, a concentration of positive charges accumulates in and on all conductive objects below the cloud. Since negative charges closer to the clouds are most efficiently repelled by the negative charges of the cloud, positive charges tend to accumulate at the top of the highest objects on the ground. In most cases that means high ground, trees, communication towers, and aerial power, telephone, and cable TV lines. It could also be you—if you are standing out in the open and are the tallest object in the area. Example: you are out playing golf and standing in the middle of the fairway.

Homes are rarely hit by lightning. When it does occur, the lightning most often takes the path of least resistance to the ground. Generally, the path of least resistance to ground in a home would include large conductive systems like the plumbing pipes, electrical wiring network, or telephone and cable TV lines, all of which are directly grounded to the Earth.

The U.S. National Safety Council reports that your odds of dying from a lightning strike during a lifetime are 1 in 126,158, and the least probable event in a list of multiple causes for death, including heart disease and cancer (1:7), assault by a firearm (1:106), and automobile accidents (1:108). This information suggests that being hit by lightning is rather unlikely. However, we recommend that you follow standard lightning safety guidelines as directed by U.S. National Weather Service (or the weather service authority in your country) if you live in a lightning-prone area. And if so, disconnect your Earthing system and don't use it during lightning and thunderstorms.

APPENDIX C

Caution:
Earthing and Medication

Most doctors have not yet heard about Earthing or don't know just how significantly it can influence the body's physiology.

For this reason, if you desire to incorporate Earthing into your daily routine and are under the care of a doctor, it is important to have a discussion with your doctor first. Earthing can influence how you feel and your medical test results and may possibly require adjustment of your medication.

Doctors have the best interests of patients at heart, so our advice is to always follow your caregiver's advice. He or she may say no to Earthing because of unfamiliarity with it or may be open to it provided there is close monitoring of medications and reporting of any unusual reactions.

In this context, medication requires special consideration, such as in the following situations:

- **Blood thinners/anticoagulants.** Earthing has a blood-thinning effect, raising the possibility of a compounded effect—and too much blood thinning—from the combination of Earthing and medication. You need to monitor your blood carefully and above all consult with your doctor.

  Steve Sinatra brings up this point: "Years ago as a practicing cardiologist in Connecticut, I often found myself having to reduce the level of warfarin (Coumadin) for patients coming back to their homes after snowbirding in Florida over the winter months. Their blood coagulability had changed. I thought it was simply a result of going from warm weather to cold weather. I was wrong. I didn't know anything about Earthing back then. I now know that the reason for the change was because they were going barefoot for many hours during the day and

273

swimming in the ocean or in concrete pools. They were grounding themselves! In the process, they were thinning their blood naturally."

- **Glucose control medication.** Regulation of blood sugar may improve with Earthing. If you take glucose control medication, monitor your glucose and check with your doctor to see if a medication reduction is in order.

- **Thyroid medication.** Earthing influences thyroid function, so if you are on thyroid medication you may begin to feel symptoms of over-medication. Talk to your doctor.

- **Anti-inflammatories.** Earthing reduces inflammation. If you take an anti-inflammatory medication, monitor your dosage with your doctor.

- **Multiple medications.** Many individuals take multiple medications. In such situations, we strongly recommend not starting Earthing without approval of one's physician. An overdose situation could develop related to one or more medications, and symptoms of overdose could appear. For somebody taking a single medication, or perhaps two, such symptoms may be apparent and easily remedied by consulting with one's doctor and reducing dosage. When multiple medications are involved, the situation is more complex. Multiple interactions could occur as different medications affect each other.

MONITOR YOURSELF

For those of you on any critical medication, decide first with your health-care giver about grounding yourself. If you decide to do it, try it for shorter periods—for a half hour or an hour—in the beginning by walking barefoot in the park or your backyard.

Slowly increase your Earthing time and monitor your situation carefully, including how you feel. Watch for signs of medication overdose. Ground with caution, and under the watchful eye of your physician.

Whether you walk barefoot on the ground outside, or eventually ground yourself indoors for many hours with an Earthing system, we want you to have the best and safest experience possible. Remember that Earthing indoors on conductive sheets, mats, or with bands and patches is the equivalent of being barefoot outdoors on the ground.

The Earthing Institute

www.earthinginstitute.net

Visit our site—Earthing's official information website—to read about the newest developments and studies regarding Earthing, as well as the growing collection of articles, videos, and feedback from around the world. You will also find answers to frequently asked questions about Earthing.

Symptom Checklist and Progress Log

To assess how grounding may be helping you, list any common symptoms you have in the column on the left. In the second column, make a note of the severity of the problem. If the symptom is pain, for instance, rate the pain on a scale of 0 to 10. Then rate the condition or symptom one week and one month after grounding. You may also want to keep track of key medical tests the same way.

OBSERVATIONS			
CONDITION/ SYMPTOM	PRE- GROUNDING	1 WEEK AFTER GROUNDING	1 MONTH AFTER GROUNDING

Earthing in Earlier Times and Indigenous Cultures

The physiological effects of grounding the human body have been documented only recently, yet physical contact with the ground has been understood by cultures throughout history in terms of connectedness or attunement with the spirit of the Earth.

What is not clear to us are these questions:

- To what degree was there understanding that this contact had specific healing properties?

- How was such understanding applied therapeutically or preventively?

Finding specific references is challenging, particularly since past cultures typically lived barefoot or used conductive animal hides for footwear and bedding. Keep in mind that when the body perspires, the moisture creates a channel of conductivity that permeates the hide. So either used as footwear or for sleeping, such natural material would allow the Earth's electrons to be transferred into the body. Thus, most cultures would have been routinely grounded to the planet's surface electrical charge, even though there was likely no awareness of the dynamics of this contact.

Being thus connected in ordinary daily life would have been sufficient to keep chronic inflammation and many typical modern diseases at bay, as well as to create other health benefits we attribute to Earthing. Earlier cultures would probably not have known the effects of being disconnected with the Earth, as they didn't have many options to be insulated other than time spent living or sleeping in elevated structures made from wood. Stone or dirt floors would have been conductive.

If you have any expertise about how grounding was utilized specifically for health purposes in the past, or even in contemporary indigenous cultures, kindly contact us at info@earthinginstitute.net.

Meanwhile, we hope you will find the following articles on past barefoot and grounding practices of interest.

AFGHANISTAN'S BAREFOOT WARRIORS

Thanks to Faizullah Kakar, Ph.D., Minister for Advising the President on Health and Education Affairs in Afghanistan, and a former official in the World Health Organization, we have learned about a historical group of warriors in the Kandahar region of his country who conducted their warfare activities barefoot.

The story, as Dr. Kakar tells it, goes back to the early eighteenth century when hardy and outnumbered Afghan rebels repeatedly fought off the powerful occupying armies of neighboring Persia and established an independent kingdom.

"Historians usually focus on the character of the leaders, but little attention is paid to the soldiers who do the actual fighting," he related. "Even less frequent is the historical focus on the physical and psychological factors that bring success to an army. Who were the men that liberated Kandahar and later established the current state called Afghanistan some 300 years ago?

"They were called the Lashkar-i-Pai-loochaan, 'the barefoot army.' Armed with a yearning for freedom, the people of Kandahar are well known for their bravery. Their mistreatment by outside rulers and an invading army enraged them and motivated them to struggle for freedom. The leaders had strict criteria for new recruits. Volunteer newcomers had to pass tests of loyalty, hardiness, and fighting skills to qualify. One of the physical requirements was to be able to live and fight barefoot on the scorching hot rocks in the summer and on freezing snow in the winter.

"I wonder," he said, "how the barefoot practice contributed to their stamina and resistance against severe weather conditions?"

Dr. Kakar's question raises good questions. In past times, soldiers and warriors surely conducted their military activities barefoot or with conductive footwear made of hides. They slept on the ground. How did these practices contribute to stamina, resistance, strength, and ability to heal from battle wounds? These are questions we can only speculate about.

We know that connection to the Earth improves circulation, energy, and healing. Clint Ober makes this observation: "If I work barefoot on a concrete floor or outdoors, I can work longer with more energy. As soon as I put shoes on, I can't go very long. It's the energy from the Earth keeping me more alert and energetic. We evolved on this energy. Think of the Kenyan and Ethiopian barefoot runners, and Tarahumara people of northwestern Mexico who run great distances barefoot."

In today's Afghanistan, according to Dr. Kakar, the "barefoot people" of Kandahar have a reputation as being the healthiest segment of the country's population. They also have a reputation as outstanding wrestlers. They still walk and work barefoot, he says.

"We also have more than 2 million nomads in Afghanistan," he adds, "and each spring, whenever new grass sprouts, they take their shoes off and walk on wet, green grass. This centuries-old tradition says that the practice is good for the eyes. In northern Afghanistan, especially in the province of Balkh, the people have a tradition called *pai-kubee*. It entails stomping on wet grass with bare feet in the early springtime in the belief that this is good for health."

As far as his own connection with the Earth is concerned, Dr. Kakar told us that since grounding himself regularly in 2011 he has experienced improved energy, deeper sleep, and elimination of aches and pains. He also told us about his niece who reported relief from headaches and low energy after she started Earthing. What really impressed him, he said, is that when she moved to another residence, where she was not able to ground herself, the headaches returned.

Dr. Kakar describes himself as an "Earthing ambassador" and has spread the word in Afghanistan among his colleagues, the media, and medical students. In 2013, he told us that some government officials were now walking barefoot on the grass in their yards.

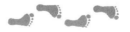

ADOLF JUST AND "EARTH POWER"

*"In all cases, and in all diseases, man can recover and again
become happy only by a true return to nature: man must
today strenuously endeavor, in his mode of living, to heed again
the voice of nature, and thus choose the food that nature has laid
before him from the beginning, and to bring himself again
into the relation with water, light and air, earth, etc.,
that nature originally designed for him."*

—ADOLF JUST, *RETURN TO NATURE! THE TRUE NATURAL
METHOD OF HEALING AND LIVING*, 1903

In the late 1800s, a natural health movement emerged in Germany. One
leading figure was Adolf Just (1859–1936), a pioneer of naturopathy, who
founded a famous sanatorium (still in business) in the Harz Mountains.
His work was said to have influenced Mahatma Gandhi.

Just's healing routines included a vegetarian diet, the use of clay packs
applied to the skin, special "porous" clothing, the avoidance of alcohol
and smoking, and an emphasis on walking barefoot and sleeping on the
ground. His activity drew considerable international attention and inspired
naturopathic movements in the United States and elsewhere.

In his book *Return to Nature!* Just placed significant attention on what
he describes as "Earth power."

"As long as man wore no shoes or clothes," he wrote, "he was always
in direct touch with the Earth, both when he moved and when he rested.
Such a close connection of man with the Earth is therefore the intention
of nature. It corresponds, moreover, to a holy, inviolable law of nature, the
transgression of which will always sternly be avenged."

Just had become increasingly convinced "of the great curative effect" of
barefoot contact with the Earth. "The feet are in a certain sense for man
what the roots are for plants. Man draws vital energy and strength out of
the Earth through his feet."

Just had drawn inspiration from a rural Bavarian parish priest named
Sebastian Kneipp, who had become somewhat of a healing celebrity. In
an 1893 book entitled *My Water Cure*, Father Kneipp described various
ways in which people could apply water for healing purposes. He also

extolled the virtues of walking barefoot. It was the "simplest and most natural practice for bracing the system," he said.

Could not this barefoot effect be expanded "on behalf of man in a still greater degree?" Just wondered. That question inspired him to recommend that patients sleep under quilts on the ground.

"They were thereby brought closer to the Earth during sleep," he wrote. "This was at once felt as a gain; sleeping became pleasanter and was more invigorating. But soon the patients lay down on the soft grass entirely naked, even without a shirt. They soon broke out in enthusiastic exclamations over the wonderful effect of the Earth upon the body during the night's rest. The opinion was often expressed that *all* diseases, but especially the score of serious nervous troubles of our age, would entirely lose their terrors if only sleeping and lying on the Earth at night once became customary in the curing of diseases. It is indeed a fact that the effect, which the forces of the Earth have upon man during the night, is quite incredible.

"By sleeping on the ground, consequently, more than by anything else, the entire body is aroused from its lethargy to a new manifestation of vital energy, so that it can now effectively remove old morbid matter and masses of old faeces from the intestines, and receive a sensation of new health, new life, and new unthought-of vigor and strength.

"Whether it is because the body at night, especially during sleep, is lying perfectly quiet, or because the influence of the Earth on the body is more powerful at night than in the day time, the fact certainly is that one does not experience the extraordinary curative effect of the Earth nearly as much in going barefooted . . . as at night."

Just observed that the first few nights on the ground might be rough, but "after that, and sometimes even in cases of protracted and obstinate insomnia, a long, exceedingly refreshing and strengthening sleep will set in. But generally most persons will soon begin to sleep less and less . . . and (yet) the brighter, fresher and stronger will they feel the next day."

After a few nights, his patients were typically "attracted to their bed on the ground, and strongly refused to tolerate anything under them. In rainy nights I was often concerned about having the patients come into the huts to sleep, so that the quilts should not get so wet, but it was with difficulty that I could induce the sick people to leave the ground. Soon, also, the hardness of lying on the ground is no longer felt. Nor need we fear that the Earth is too cold at night to lie on entirely naked under covers; we shall only experience the sensation of a delightful coolness."

For beginners, he recommended lying naked on the ground under covers only on warm summer nights, or in very mild spring and autumn nights.

Just sought to make his paying guests maximally comfortable and built his natural outdoor beds on a layer of sand four to eight inches. The sand could be covered with burlap or linen, he noted, "without weakening the effect of the Earth power."

Just strongly disapproved of modern beds. "The defectiveness of beds will be felt as long as men shall decline to sleep on the bed which kind nature herself has created for her creatures," he wrote, "and which she has endowed with a magic power by which man receives a greater enjoyment of life."

To promote the idea of sleeping on the ground to patients, Just often referred to animals in the wild. He wrote: "Hares and deer, when they prepare their lair, carefully remove all leaves, bits of wood, etc. The fox and badger drag many things into their dens, but their resting place is kept perfectly free. It is always on the bare ground. They evidently do this to be more directly in touch with the Earth, so that the forces of the Earth may exert the strongest possible effect. The animals do not scrape together grass, leaves, wood, and the like for their beds—birds only do this in order to prepare a warm nest for hatching. It is a very striking fact that the animals of the woods always remove all the wood and leaves, and even the snow, so as to make an entirely bare spot on the Earth where they may lie down and rest. I once observed a domestic hog that was sick and was let out of its sty. On my advice it was left entirely alone, so that it might do what it wanted to. It went into the vegetable garden, grubbed itself somewhat into the ground in a cabbage bed, and remained quietly lying there. After a few days it returned and—was perfectly well."

Just didn't expect people to rush to his ideas, but he urged them to consider at least going barefooted "excepting a few very cold weeks in winter . . . without ever feeling the custom as a torture or a burden, but rather as the greatest delight and pleasure. Going barefooted is no asceticism, but an augmentation of the enjoyment of life. For the Earth has her son again, as soon as man goes barefooted, and can again shower on him fresh health and true happiness."

GEORGE STARR WHITE, M.D.:
LESS GROUNDED, LESS HEALTH

George Starr White, M.D., Ph.D. (1866–1956), a prodigious and prolific physician, attracted considerable attention and controversy because of his outspoken advocacy of natural healing methods and criticism of medical dogma during the late 1800s and first part of the twentieth century. Among the ideas he promoted in his many books and lectures was to apply the Earth's energy for healing and better sleep. He often recommended to patients with sleeping difficulties to ground themselves in bed with a bare copper wire placed under the bottom sheet. The other end of the wire was attached or soldered to a ground rod outside, a water or gas pipe, or a steam radiator.

In *Cosmo-Electro Culture for Land and Man*, a book he published in 1940, he contended that the less humans lived grounded—connected in some manner to the Earth—the more unhealthy they became. He learned over many decades, he said, "that all animals and humans who lived naturally were always directly or indirectly grounded. So-called civilization has attempted to make it possible for humans, as well as some animals, to live not grounded, but the results are consequently bad."

THE HADZABE—A BAREFOOT WAY OF LIFE

Iowa psychotherapist-anthropologist Geral Blanchard, L.P.C., is author of *Ancient Ways* (2011), a book about indigenous healing traditions around the world. He has studied and lived with many native populations, including the Bushmen of Africa. He shared the following information with us:

"The vast majority of Bushmen have been assimilated into the dominant African melting pot culture and so there are but a few thousand that still live on the Earth, hunting and healing as they did for tens of thousands of years. These individuals include the Hadzabe in northwest Tanzania, whom I have visited a number of times. They have the closest link to the Earth I have ever seen in my travels and studies. They appear to be quintessential spokespeople for Earthing.

"They sit and walk on the Earth all day long. They are hunter-gatherers; one of the extremely rare foraging groups remaining on Earth. They some-

times sleep under the partial cover of a thatched hut, but at most are separated from the Earth only by a woven mat made from vegetation or by
an impala hide. By day, they are seated with each other directly on the
Earth, talking and resting, between hunts.

"This near-extinct group, like so many other Bushmen, sometimes wear
sandals made from spent motorcycle tires found in their meanderings, or
from animal hides, or plastic versions donated by missionaries. Much of
the time you see sandals scattered on the ground and both adults and children walking around barefoot.

"The Hadzabe connection to the land is virtually unbroken; they avoid
civilization and entering into any steel-covered buildings because they
believe such structures are not healthy in part because they are not in connection with the Earth. In fact, most of them won't let their children be
taken to government schools as the children are kept in sheltered structures with metal roofs.

"Government studies of the Hadzabe reveal that their health is better
than most other rural Africans, the majority of whom are agricultural and
pastoral, but most of whom, unlike the Hadzabe, have access to Western-
style health care. Simply put, the Hadzabe receive little or no organized
health care, primarily because they don't get ill. Interestingly, each individual knows enough about natural remedies that a doctor/shaman is not
part of their culture; they are walking compendiums of plant medicines
who simply take care of themselves. Everyone is efficacious in all aspects
of life, including being his or her own 'doctor.' The Hadzabe diet doesn't
lend itself to all the maladies related to obesity. They have none.

"The studies speak of extremely good eyesight, hearing, and teeth. There
appears to be no cancer. Women experience few effects of menopause.
There are no reports of issues such as hot flashes. Menstrual periods are
shorter than in the West, only about three days in length; the flow is not
as copious. Women remain hardy into their seventies. Sterility is rare. Sex-
ually transmitted diseases are comparatively uncommon when compared
to neighboring tribes that live indoors. Injury and death are usually the
result of accidents: cuts, falls, animal encounters, including snakebites.
Infant mortality during the first year is high, about 21 percent.

"Heading south into South Africa, Botswana, and Namibia, you find
other groups of Bushman distantly separated from their northern coun-

terparts long, long ago. Unlike the Hadzabe, the southern Bushman—the Kalahari Desert Kung, San, and Ju'hoansi peoples—practice so-called 'trance dances.' They are said to be masters of using 'boiling energy,' or *num*, as it is called, for healing. Num is the Earth's energy and is regarded as a spiritual energy that can help people cross time barriers and communicate with ancestors. Num is felt, at first, on their bare feet during all-night dancing. It moves up the entire body to the head. Legs can be seen trembling; eventually the entire body shivers and then convulses. It creates piercing heat (as if it is coming from pointed 'arrows') in the abdomen that leaves its carriers bent forward. It resides primarily in the pit of the stomach and the base of the spine. The liver and spleen are thought to heat up. An altered state develops, called *kia*, when energy reaches the brain. Rapid, shallow breathing is used to bring the num up. When you are filled with num, others want to touch you as this type of healthy energy is thought to be contagious, but a desirable spreading contagion quite the opposite of illness. They use healing touch from their fluttering hands to heal one another. During kia, with the Earth's energy filling the individual and group, amazing physical feats are possible, including handling or walking on fire, seeing inside other people's bodies with x-ray-like vision, as well as improved long-distance sight.

"Unlike many Western doctors and scientists who break the body down into separated organs, the Bushmen refer to a more holistic healing process experienced with num. Not only are they healed of their few existing ailments, perhaps more important their social ties are strengthened. Being the oldest people on Earth, they still maintain primal powers and remain 'plugged into' the Earth's natural regenerative and recalibrating forces.

"Many anthropological types, like myself, have seen enough seemingly extraordinary human abilities tapped from nature by indigenous people that it would appear the human race is atrophying in its ability to use such healing forces."

Earthing Research

Biological Studies

Chevalier G, Sinatra ST, Oschman JL, et al. "Earthing (grounding) the human body reduces blood viscosity: A major factor in cardiovascular disease." *Journal of Alternative and Complementary Medicine* 2013; 19(2): 102–110; published online at: http://online.liebertpub.com/doi/pdplus/10.1089/acm.2011.0820.

Objectives: Emerging research is revealing that direct physical contact of the human body with the surface of the earth (grounding or earthing) has intriguing effects on human physiology and health, including beneficial effects on various cardiovascular risk factors. This study examined effects of 2 hours of grounding on the electrical charge (zeta potential) on red blood cells (RBCs) and the effects on the extent of RBC clumping. *Design/interventions:* Subjects were grounded with conductive patches on the soles of their feet and the palms of their hands. Wires connected the patches to a stainless-steel rod inserted in the Earth outdoors. Small fingertip pinprick blood samples were placed on microscope slides and an electric field was applied to them. Electrophoretic mobility of the RBCs was determined by measuring terminal velocities of the cells in video recordings taken through a microscope. RBC aggregation was measured by counting the numbers of clustered cells in each sample. *Settings/location:* Each subject sat in a comfortable reclining chair in a soundproof experiment room with the lights dimmed or off. *Subjects:* Ten healthy adult subjects were recruited by word-of-mouth. *Results:* Earthing or grounding increased zeta potentials in all samples by an average of 2.70 and significantly reduced RBC aggregation. *Conclusions:* Grounding increases the surface charge on RBCs and thereby reduces blood viscosity and clumping. Grounding appears to be one of the simplest and yet most profound interventions for helping reduce cardiovascular risk and cardiovascular events.

Sokal P, Jastrzebski Z, Jaskulska E, et al. "Differences in blood urea and creatinine concentrations in earthed and unearthed subjects during cycling exercise and recovery." *Evidence-Based Complementary and Alternative Medicine* 2013; published online at: http://www.hindawi.com/journals/ecam/2013/382643.

Contact of humans with the earth, either directly (e.g., with bare feet) or using a metal conductor, changes their biochemical parameters. The effects of earthing during physical exercise are unknown. This study was carried out to evaluate selected biochemical parameters in subjects who were earthed during cycling. In a double-blind crossover study, 42 participants were divided into two groups and earthed during exercise and recovery. One group was earthed in the first week during 30 minutes of cycling exercise and during recovery, and a second group was earthed in the second week. A double-blind technique was applied. Blood samples were obtained before each training session, after 15 and 30 minutes of exercise, and after 40 minutes of recovery. Significantly lower blood urea levels were observed in subjects earthed during exercise and relaxation. These significant differences were noted in both groups earthed at the beginning of exercise ($P < 0.0001$), after 15 ($P < 0.0001$) and 30 minutes ($P < 0.0001$) of exercise, and after 40 minutes of relaxation ($P < 0.0001$). Creatinine concentrations in earthed subjects during exercise were unchanged. *Conclusions:* Earthing during exercise lowers blood urea concentrations and may inhibit hepatic protein catabolism or increase renal urea excretion. Exertion under earthing may result in a positive protein balance.

Chevalier G, Sinatra ST, Oschman JL, et al. "Earthing: Health implications of reconnecting the human body to the Earth's surface electrons." *Journal of Environmental and Public Health* 2012; published online at: www.hindawi.com/journals/jeph/2012/291541.

Environmental medicine generally addresses environmental factors with a negative impact on human health. However, emerging scientific research has revealed a surprisingly positive and overlooked environmental factor on health: direct physical contact with the vast supply of electrons on the surface of the Earth. Modern lifestyle separates humans from such contact. The research suggests that this disconnect may be a major contributor to physiological dysfunction and unwellness. Reconnection with the Earth's electrons has been found to promote intriguing physiological changes and subjective reports of well-being. Earthing (or grounding) refers to the discovery of benefits—including better sleep and reduced pain—from walking barefoot outside or sitting, working, or sleeping indoors connected to conductive systems that transfer the Earth's electrons from the ground into the body. This paper reviews the earthing research and the potential of earthing as a simple and easily accessed global modality of significant clinical importance.

Sokal K, Sokal P. "Earthing the human organism influences bioelectrical processes." *Journal of Alternative and Complementary Medicine* 2012; 18(3): 229–234; published online at: http://online.liebertpub.com/doi/abs/10.1089/acm.2010.0683.

Objectives: This article describes interaction of the Earth's mass—electrolytic conductor on the electrical environment of human organism—aqueous environment and skeleton. In this environment, bioelectrical, and bioenergetical processes take place. *Methods and subjects:* Measurements of electric potential on tongue, teeth, nails, and in venous blood in subjects earthed and unearthed were conducted in Faraday's cage with the use of an electrometer placed outside the cage. Measurements were performed in subjects in lying position and in movements of standing up and lying down. *Results:* In the unearthed human organism in the lying position, electric potential measured in examined points is around 0 mV. Contact of the Earth by a copper conductor with a moistened surface of the human body evokes a rapid decrease of electrostatic potential on the body and in venous blood to the value of approximately –200 mV. This effect is immediate and general. Interruption of contact with the Earth causes a rapid return of the potential to its initial values in examined points. Changes in electric potential measured in venous blood and on mucosal membrane of the tongue reflect alterations in electric potential of the aqueous, electrical environment. Up-and-down movement of the insulated human organism causes transient changes in potential in the human electrical environment. During the same movement, values of potential in the electrical environment of an earthed human body remain constant. *Conclusions:* These results indicate that up-and-down movement and the elimination of potentials in the electrical environment of the human organism by the Earth's mass may play a fundamental role in regulation of bioelectrical and bioenergetical processes. The Earth's electromagnetohydrodynamic potential is responsible for this phenomenon.

Sokal P, Sokal K. "The neuromodulative role of Earthing." *Medical Hypotheses* 2011; 77(5): 824–826; published online at www.medical-hypotheses.com/article/ S0306-9877(11)00364-1/abstract.

Neuromodulation is a process of inhibition, stimulation, modification, and regulation or therapeutic alteration of activity, electrically and chemically in the peripheral, central or autonomic nervous systems. Direct electric current or electric field alternates the function of nervous system. Coupling the human organism with the Earth directly or via a wire conductor changes the electric potential not only on the surface of the body but also inside it, changing the potential of electric environment of the human organism. Earthing refers to a direct contact with the Earth with bare feet, or contact with the Earth with the use of conductive wire attached to the human body during sleeping, or daily activities. During earthing this electric potential equals with the electric potential of the Earth and the value of it depends on location, time, atmospheric conditions, moisture of the surface of the Earth. The earthing, which changes the density of negative charge in the electric environment of the human body, influences physiological processes. Our medical hypothesis states that contact with the Earth (earthing) directly or via a conductive wire plays a role as a neuromodulative factor, probably primary, which enables the nervous system to be better adapted to the demands of the organism and ambient environment. It helps to restore the natural, electrical status of the electrical environment of the organism and thus the nervous system. Earthing generates immediate changes in electroencephalography (EEG), surface electromyography (SEMG), and somato-sensory evoked potentials (SSEPs). We hypothesize that earthing through its complex action on the bioelectrical environment of human organism and alternations in electrolyte concentrations regulates correct functioning of the nervous system. Earthing significantly influences the electrical activity of the brain.

Chevalier G, Sinatra ST. "Emotional stress, heart rate variability, grounding, and improved autonomic tone: Clinical applications." *Integrative Medicine: A Clinician's Journal* 2011; 10(3): 16–21; published online at http://74.63.154.231/here/wp-content/uploads/2013/06/Chevalier-Sinatra-HRV-Paper-2011.pdf.

Over the last few years, the utilization of integrative biophysics for medical application has been increasing in popularity. Grounding or earthing is the oldest and most basic form of natural bioelectric potential that supports physiological and electrophysiological changes in the body. Since previous investigations have shown that grounding profoundly affects skin conductance within seconds, we hypothesized that grounding may also improve heart rate variability (HRV). In this study of 27 final participants, grounded subjects had improvements in HRV that go beyond basic relaxation (P<.01). Since improved HRV has such a positive impact on cardiovascular status, it is suggested that simple grounding techniques be utilized as a basic integrative strategy in supporting the cardiovascular system, especially under situations of heightened autonomic tone (i.e., when the sympathetic nervous system is more activated than the parasympathetic nervous system).

Sokal K, Sokal P. "Earthing the human body influences physiologic processes." *Journal of Alternative and Complementary Medicine* 2011; 17(4): 301–308; published online at http://74.63.154.231/here/wpcontent/uploads/2013/06/Sokal_Sokal_earthing_influence_physiology-2010.pdf.

Objectives: This study was designed to answer the question: Does the contact of the human organism with the Earth via a copper conductor affect physiologic processes? *Subjects and experiments:* Five (5) experiments are presented: Experiment 1–Effect of earthing on calcium-phosphate homeostasis and serum concentrations of iron (N=84 participants); Experiment 2–Effect of earthing on serum concentrations of electrolytes (N=28); Experiment 3–Effect of earthing on thyroid function (N=12); Experiment 4–Effect of earthing on glucose concentration (N=12); Experiment 5–Effect of earthing on immune response to vaccine (N=32). Subjects were divided into two groups. One (1) group of people was earthed, while the second group remained without contact with the Earth. Blood and urine samples were examined. *Results:* Earthing of an electrically insulated human organism during night rest causes lowering of serum concentrations of iron, ionized calcium, inorganic phosphorus, and reduction of renal excretion of calcium and phosphorus. Earthing during night rest decreases free tri-iodothyronine and increases free thyroxine and thyroid-stimulating hormone. The continuous earthing of the human body decreases blood glucose in patients with diabetes. Earthing decreases sodium, potassium, magnesium, iron, total protein, and albumin concentrations, while the levels of transferrin, ferritin, and globulins $\alpha1$, $\alpha2$, β, and γ increase. These results are statistically significant. *Conclusions:* Earthing the human body influences human physiologic processes. This influence is observed during night relaxation and during physical activity. Effect of the earthing on calcium-phosphate homeostasis is the opposite of that which occurs in states of weightlessness. It also increases the activity of catabolic processes. It may be the primary factor regulating endocrine and nervous systems.

Brown D, Chevalier G, Hill M. "Pilot study on the effect of grounding on delayed onset muscle soreness." *Journal of Alternative and Complementary Medicine* 2010; 16(3): 265–273; published online at http://74.63.154.231/here/wpcontent/uploads/2013/ 06/ Brown_Chevalier_Hill_earthing_delayed_muscle_2010.pdf.

Objectives: The purpose of this pilot study was to determine whether there are markers that can be used to study the effects of grounding on delayed-onset muscle soreness (DOMS). *Design and subjects:* Eight healthy subjects were exposed to an eccentric exercise that caused DOMS in gastrocnemius muscles [calf muscle] of both legs. Four subjects were grounded with electrode patches and patented conductive sheets connected to the earth. Four (4) control subjects were treated identically, except that the grounding systems were not connected to the earth. *Outcome measures:* Complete blood counts, blood chemistry, enzyme chemistry, serum and saliva cortisols, magnetic resonance imaging and spectroscopy and pain levels were taken at the same time of day before the eccentric exercise and 24, 48, and 72 hours afterward. Parameters consistently differing by 10% or more, normalized to baseline, were considered worthy of further study. *Results:* Parameters that differed by these criteria included white blood cell counts, bilirubin, creatine kinase, phosphocreatine/inorganic phosphate ratios, glycerolphosphorylcholine, phosphorylcholine, the visual analogue pain scale, and pressure measurements on the right gastrocnemius. *Conclusions:* In a pilot study, grounding the body to the earth alters measures of immune system activity and pain. Since this is the first intervention that appears to speed recovery from DOMS, the pilot provides a basis for a larger study.

Chevalier G. **"Changes in pulse rate, respiratory rate, blood oxygenation, perfusion index, skin conductance and their variability induced during and after grounding human subjects for forty minutes."** *Journal of Alternative and Complementary Medicine* 2010; 16(1): 81–87; published online at http://74.63.154.231/here/wpcontent/ uploads/2013/06/Chevalier_earthing_pulse_rate-2010.pdf.

Objectives: Previous studies have shown that grounding produces quantifiable physiologic changes. This study was set up to reproduce and expand earlier electrophysiologic and physiologic parameters measured immediately after grounding with improved methodology and state-of-the-art equipment. *Design and subjects:* A multi-parameter double-blind experiment was conducted with 14 men and 14 women (age range: 18–80) in relatively good health. Subjects were screened for health problems using a commonly used health questionnaire. They were seated in a comfortable recliner and measured during 2-hour grounding sessions, leaving time for signals to stabilize before, during, and after grounding (40 minutes for each period). Sham 2-hour grounding sessions were also recorded with the same subjects as controls. *Outcome measures:* This report presents results for 5 of the 18 parameters measured. The parameters reported here are: skin conductance (SC), blood oxygenation (BO), respiratory rate (RR), pulse rate (PR), and perfusion index (PI). *Settings/location:* This study was performed in a rented facility in Encinitas, California. The facility was chosen in a quiet area for its very low electromagnetic noise. *Results:* For each session, statistical analyses were performed on four 10-minute segments: before and after grounding (sham grounding for control session), and before and after ungrounding (sham ungrounding). There was an immediate decrease in SC at grounding and an immediate increase at ungrounding on all subjects. RR increased during grounding, and the effect lasted after ungrounding. RR variance increased immediately after grounding then decreased. BO variance decreased during grounding, followed by a dramatic increase after ungrounding. PR and PI variances increased toward the end of the grounding period, and this change persisted after ungrounding. *Conclusions:* These results warrant further research to determine how grounding affects the body. Grounding could become important for relaxation, health maintenance, and disease prevention.

Chevalier G, Mori K. "The effect of earthing on human physiology (part II): Electrodermal measurements." *Subtle Energy and Energy Medicine* 2007; 18(3): 11–34; published online at http://journals.sfu.ca/seemj/index.php/seemj/article/view/9/7.

The human body evolved while living in direct electrical contact (electrically grounded) with the earth. The question that arises is: Does loss of electrical contact with the earth affect human physiology? This double-blind study was designed to address this question by measuring several electrophysiological parameters of the body. Subjects were assigned to an experimental group that was grounded to the earth after a 28-minute baseline recording. Grounding the body (earthing) was achieved by placing electrode patches on the soles of the feet and connecting them to a conductive cable that was attached to a metal rod planted in the earth. The total recording time was 56 minutes. *The control group was not grounded but "sham grounded."* Part 1 of this study presented results from measurements taken with clinical biofeedback equipment. This paper presents results obtained on Jing-Well points using the SSVP (Single Square Voltage Pulse) method. With the SSVP method we were able to corroborate results presented in our first paper with the biofeedback system. The SSVP method results are that grounding the body produces a reduction in tension (relaxation) of the internal organs and a reduction in inflammation. We also postulated that the body was developed to take advantage of the contact with the earth through the feet by developing a system of distribution of electrons through the kidney meridian at kidney 1. The present findings are consistent with the results of our previous study, which concluded that grounded subjects experienced a reduction in stress and a normalization of the functioning of the autonomic nervous system after earthing.

Chevalier G, Mori K, Oschman, JL. "The effect of Earthing (grounding) on human physiology." *European Biology and Bioelectromagnetics*, January 31, 2006; 600–621; published online at http://74.63.154.231/here/wp-content/uploads/2013/06/The-effect-of-earthing-on-human-physiology-Part-1-2006.pdf.

Previous research showed that connecting the human body to the earth during sleep normalizes circadian cortisol profiles and reduces or eliminates various subjectively reported symptoms, including sleep dysfunction, pain, and stress. We, therefore, hypothesized that earthing might also influence other aspects of physiology. Fifty-eight healthy adult subjects (30 controls) participated in a double-blind pilot study. Earthing was accomplished with a conductive adhesive patch placed on the sole of each foot. An earthing cord led outdoors to a rod driven into the earth. A biofeedback system recorded electrophysiological and physiological parameters. Upon earthing, about half the experimental subjects showed an abrupt, almost instantaneous change in root mean square (rms) values of electroencephalograms (EEG) from the left hemisphere (but not the right hemisphere) and all of them presented an abrupt change in rms values of surface electromyograms (SEMGs) from right and left upper trapezius muscles. Signal variance in rms muscle potentials also increased significantly. Earthing decreased blood volume pulse (BVP) in 19 of 22 experimental subjects (p < 0.001) and in 8 of 30 controls (p ≅ 0.1, not significant); heart rate (HR) was not affected. From these results, it appears that earthing the human body has significant effects on electrophysiological properties of the brain and musculature, on the blood volume pulse, and on the noise and stability of electrophysiological recordings. Taken together, the changes in EEG, EMG, and BVP suggest reductions in overall stress levels and tensions, and a shift in autonomic balance upon earthing.

Ghaly M, Teplitz D. "The biologic effects of grounding the human body during sleep as measured by cortisol levels and subjective reporting of sleep, pain, and stress. *Journal of Alternative and Complementary Medicine* 2004; 10(5): 767–776; published online at http://74.63.154.231/here/wpcontent/uploads/2013/06/Ghaly_Teplitz_cortisol_study_2004.pdf.

Objectives: Diurnal cortisol secretion levels were measured and circadian cortisol profiles were evaluated in a pilot study conducted to test the hypothesis that grounding the human body to earth during sleep will result in quantifiable changes in cortisol. It was also hypothesized that grounding the human body would result in changes in sleep, pain, and stress (anxiety, depression, irritability), as measured by subjective reporting. *Subjects and Interventions:* Twelve subjects with complaints of sleep dysfunction, pain, and stress were grounded to earth during sleep for 8 weeks in their own beds using a conductive mattress pad. Saliva tests were administered to establish pregrounding baseline cortisol levels. Levels were obtained at 4-hour intervals for a 24-hour period to determine the circadian cortisol profile. Cortisol testing was repeated at week 6. Subjective symptoms of sleep dysfunction, pain, and stress were reported daily throughout the 8-week test period. *Results:* Measurable improvements in diurnal cortisol profiles were observed, with cortisol levels significantly reduced during nighttime sleep. Subjects' 24-hour circadian cortisol profiles showed a trend toward normalization. Subjectively reported symptoms, including sleep dysfunction, pain, and stress, were reduced or eliminated in nearly all subjects. *Conclusions:* Results indicate that grounding the human body to earth ("earthing") during sleep reduces nighttime levels of cortisol and resynchronizes cortisol hormone secretion more in alignment with the natural 24-hour circadian rhythm profile. Changes were most apparent in females. Furthermore, subjective reporting indicates that grounding the human body to earth during sleep improves sleep and reduces pain and stress.

Earthing Electrical Study

Applewhite R. "The effectiveness of a conductive patch and a conductive bed pad in reducing induced human body voltage via the application of earth ground." *European Biology and Bioelectromagnetics* 2005; 1: 23–40; published online at http:// 74.63.154.231/here/wpcontent/uploads/2013/06/Applewhite_earthing_ body_voltage_2005.pdf.

Voltage induced on a human body by capacitive coupling to the external environment was measured using a high-impedance measurement head. The body was then earth grounded by means of a conductive patch and a conductive bed pad. Each method reduced the coupled 60 Hz mains voltage by a factor of at least 70. This result, along with the measurement of the voltage drop across an in-line resistance in the conductive patch provided evidence of a simplified electrical network model of the human body.

Selected Bibliography

Chapter 2

Franceschi C, Bonafe M, Valensin S, et al. "Inflamm-aging: an evolutionary perspective on immunosenescence." *Annals New York Academy of Sciences* 2006; 908: 244–254.

Gorman C, and Park A. "The fires within." *Time* Feb 23, 2004; 38–46.

Meggs W. *The Inflammation Cure.* New York: McGraw-Hill, 2004.

Oschman JL. "Our place in Nature: reconnecting with the Earth for better sleep." *Journal of Alternative and Complementary Medicine* 2003; 10(5): 735–36.

Suckling EE. *The Living Battery—An Introduction to Bioelectricity.* New York: Macmillan, 1964.

Chapter 3

Bach JF. "Why is the incidence of autoimmune diseases increasing in the modern world?" *Endocrine Abstracts* 2008; 16(S3): 1.

Bower B. "Slumber's unexplored landscape." *Science News Online* Sept 25, 1999.

Gish OH. "The natural electric currents in the Earth. *Scientific Monthly* 1936; 43(1): 47–57.

International Inflammation (in-FLAME) Network summary report from 2012 workshop. "Risk factors, pathways and early preventive strategies targeting inflammation as a common antecedent of NCDs"; http://wun.ac.uk/sites/default/files/in-flame_ workshop_report_may_2012.pdf.

Max Planck Institutes. Research cited in *Energy Medicine: The Scientific Basis* by James L. Oschman (Churchill Livingstone, 2000): 101.

Stein R. "Is modern life ravaging our immune systems?" *Washington Post* Mar 4, 2008.

Tavera M. "The sacred mission"(translated by George Verdon). *ESD Journal* 2008; www.esdjournal.com/articles/sacredmission.htm.

Williams ER and Heckman SJ. "The local diurnal variation of cloud electrification and the global diurnal variation of negative charge on the earth." *Journal of Geophysical Research* 1993; 98: 5221–5234.

Chapter 5

Cho HJ, Lavretsky H, Olmstead R, et al. "Sleep disturbance and depression recurrence in community-dwelling older adults: a prospective study." *American Journal of Psychiatry* 2008; 165(12): 1543–1550.

Ghaly M. and Teplitz D. "The biologic effects of grounding the human body during sleep as measured by cortisol levels and subjective reporting of sleep, pain and stress." *Journal of Alternative and Complementary Medicine* 2004; 10(5): 767–776.

Irwin MR, Wang M, Ribeiro D, et al. "Sleep loss activates cellular inflammatory signaling." *Biological Psychiatry* 2008; 64(6): 538–540.

Ober AC. "Grounding the human body to earth reduces chronic inflammation and related chronic pain." *ESD Journal* Jul 2003; www.esdjournal.com/articles/cober/ earth.htm.

Ober AC. "Grounding the human body to neutralize bio-electrical stress from static electricity and EMFs." *ESD Journal* Jan 2000; www.esdjournal.com/articles/cober/ ground.htm.

Simpson N and Dinges DF. "Sleep and inflammation." *Nutrition Review* 2007; 65(12, part II): S244–52.

Chapter 7

Amalu W. "A pilot study test of grounding the human body to reduce inflammation." Unpublished data.

Omoigui S. "The origin of all pain is inflammation and the inflammatory response: a unifying law of pain." *Medical Hypotheses* 2007; 69: 70–82.

Oschman JL. "Charge transfer in the living matrix." *Journal of Bodywork and Movement Therapies* 2009; 13: 215–28.

Pischinger A. *Extracellular Matrix and Ground Regulation: Basis for a Holistic Biological Medicine.* Berkeley, CA: North Atlantic Books, 2007 (revised and updated English translation of *Das System der Grundregulation: Grundlagen für eine ganzheitsbiologische Theorie der Medizin,* originally published by K.F. Haug, Heidelberg, 1975).

Ridker PM, et al. "Inflammation, aspirin, and the risk of cardiovascular-disease in apparently healthy men." *New England Journal of Medicine* 1997; 336(14): 973–979.

Ridker PM, et al. "C-reactive protein and other markers of inflammation in the prediction of cardiovascular disease in women." *New England Journal of Medicine* 2000; 342(12): 836–843.

Salvioli S, et al. "Inflamm-aging, cytokines and aging: state of the art, new hypotheses on the role of mitochondria and new perspectives from systems biology." *Current Pharmaceutical Design* 2006; 12(24): 3161–3171.

Chapter 8

Applewhite R. "The effectiveness of a conductive patch and a conductive bed pad in reducing induced human body voltage via the application of earth ground." *European Biology and Bioelectromagnetics* 2005; 1: 23–40.

Brown D, Chevalier G, Hill M. "Pilot study on the effect of grounding on delayed onset muscle soreness." *Journal of Alternative and Complementary Medicine* 2010: 16(3): 265–273.

Chevalier G, Mori K, Oschman, JL. "The effect of earthing (grounding) on human physiology." *European Biology and Bioelectromagnetics* Jan 31, 2006; 600–621.

Chevalier G, and Mori K. "The effect of earthing on human physiology (part II): electrodermal measurements." *Subtle Energy and Energy Medicine* 2007: 18(3): 11–34.

Chevalier G. "Changes in pulse rate, respiratory rate, blood oxygenation, perfusion index, skin conductance and their variability induced during and after grounding human subjects for forty minutes." *Journal of Alternative and Complementary Medicine* 2010: 16(1): 81–87.

Feynman R, Leighton RB, and Sands M. *The Feynman Lectures on Physics* (vol II). Reading, MA: Addison-Wesley Publishing, 1964: Chapter 9.

Jamiesona KS, ApSimona HM, Jamiesona SS, et al. "The effects of electric fields on charged molecules and particles in individual microenvironments." *Atmospheric Environment* 2007; 41: 5224–5235.

Ober AC. "Grounding the human body to neutralize bio-electrical stress from static electricity and EMFs." *ESD Journal* 2004; www.esdjournal.com/articles/cober /ground.htm.

Ober AC, and Coghill RW. "Does grounding the human body to earth reduce chronic inflammation and related chronic pain?" Presentation at the European Bioelectromagnetics Association Annual Meeting, November 12, 2003, Budapest, Hungary.

Oschman JL. "Can electrons act as antioxidants? a review and commentary." *Journal of Alternative and Complementary Medicine* 2007; 13(9): 955–967.

Oschman JL. "Assume a spherical cow: the role of free or mobile electrons in bodywork, energetic and movement therapies." *Journal of Bodywork and Movement Therapies* 2008; 12: 40–57.

Oschman JL, and Kessler WD. "Energy medicine and anti-aging: from fundamentals to new breakthroughs." *Anti-Aging Medical News* Winter 2008: 166–171.

Sokal K, and Sokal P. "Earthing the human body influences physiologic processes." *Journal of Alternative and Complementary Medicine* 2011; 17(4): 301–308.

Sokal K, and Sokal P. "Earthing the human organism influences bioelectrical processes." *Journal of Alternative and Complementary Medicine* 2012; 18(3): 229–234.

Sokal P, and Sokal K. "The neuromodulative role of Earthing." Medical Hypotheses 2011; 77(5): 824–826.

Chapter 9

Yang J. "No shoes? No problem." July 15, 2009; http:// www.theglobeandmail.com/ life/health/no-shoes-no-problem/article1219575.

Chapter 11

Chevalier G, and Sinatra ST. "Emotional stress, heart rate variability, grounding, and improved autonomic tone: clinical applications." *Integrative Medicine: A Clinician's Journal* 2011; 10(3): 16–21.

Chevalier G, Sinatra ST, Oschman JL, et al. "Earthing (grounding) the human body reduces blood viscosity: a major factor in cardiovascular disease. *Journal of Alternative and Complementary Medicine* 2013; 19(2): 102–110.

Fontes A, Fernandes HP, et al. "Measuring electrical and mechanical properties of red blood cells with double optical tweezers." *Journal of Biomedical Optics* 2008; 13(1): 014001.

"Global high blood pressure situation growing dire, but doesn't have to be, new health report says." *Medical News Today,* May 18, 2007; www.medicalnewstoday.com/ articles/71331.php.

Shaper AG. "Cardiovascular disease in the tropics." *British Medical Journal* 1972; 4(5831): 32–35.

Chapter 14

Sokal P, Jastrzebski Z, Jaskulska E, et al. "Differences in blood urea and creatinine concentrations in earthed and unearthed subjects during cycling exercise and recovery." *Evidence-Based Complementary and Alternative Medicine* 2013; www.hindawi .com/journals/ecam/2013/382643.

Chapter 15

Puotinen CJ. "Earth energy." *Whole Dog Journal* Jan. 2008: 17–21.

Chapter 17

Beasley JD and Swift J. "The Kellogg Report: the impact of nutrition, environment & lifestyle on the health of Americans." Annandale-on-Hudson, NY: Bard College Center, Institute of Health Policy and Practice, 1989.

Council of State Governments. "Costs of chronic diseases: what are states facing?" *Trends Alert* 2006.

Murray C, et al (U.S. Burden of Disease Collaborators). "The state of U.S. health, 1990–2010; burden of diseases, injuries, and risk factors." *Journal of American Medical Association* 2013; 310(6): 591–608.

United Nations Dept. of Economic and Social Affairs, Population Division. "World population ageing: 1950–2050"; www.un.org/esa/population/publications/world ageing19502050.

World Health Organization. "Ageing and life course: 2013 report on care and independence in older age"; www.who.int/ageing/en.

Appendix A

Fly Light Aviation Meteorology. "Atmospheric electricity"; www.auf.asn.au/meteorology/ section11.html.

Sokal K, and Sokal P. "Earthing the human organism influences bioelectrical processes." *Journal of Alternative and Complementary Medicine* 2012; 18(3): 229–234.

Appendix F

Just A. *Return to Nature! The True Natural Method of Healing and Living and the True Salvation of the Soul,* trans. from the German by Benedict Lust. New York: Volunteer Press, 1903.

White GS. *Cosmo-Electro Culture for Land and Man.* Los Angeles: self-published, 1940.

White GS. *The Finer Forces of Nature in Diagnosis and Therapy.* Originally published, 1903; reprinted Albuquerque, NM: Sun Books, 1981.

Acknowledgments

To James Oschman, Ph.D., an extraordinary biophysicist, who has exhaustively researched the science related to the healing benefits of Earthing. He was the first to scientifically explain the transfer of free electrons from the Earth's pulsating surface into the electric matrix of the human body. His investigations, hypotheses, and published papers on the subject have given solid scientific basis to a paradigm-shifting health concept. Dr. Oschman is the director of Nature's Own Research Association in Dover, New Hampshire (www.energyresearch.bizland.com) and the author of *Energy Medicine: The Scientific Basis* (Churchill Livingstone, 2000) and *Energy Medicine in Therapeutics and Human Performance* (Butterworth-Heinemann, 2003). His work explores the existence of a high-speed communication system extending throughout the human body that responds to the energetic environment. Dr. Oschman holds a Ph.D. in biological sciences from the University of Pittsburgh. He is a member of the Scientific Advisory Board of the National Foundation for Alternative Medicine in Washington, D.C.

To Gaétan Chevalier, Ph.D., visiting researcher at the Developmental and Cell Biology Department, University of California at Irvine, and the keenest of biological investigators. His experiments and findings on the bioelectrical changes brought about by grounding have opened a new frontier of electrophysiological research examining the striking differences between grounded and nongrounded human beings. Dr. Chevalier holds a Ph.D. in engineering physics from the University of Montreal. He was formerly director of research at the California Institute for Human Science.

To Polish cardiologist Karol Sokal, M.D., Ph.D., and his neurosurgeon son Pawel Sokal, M.D., Ph.D., for being ahead of all of us in the scientific exploration of the Earth's electrical field effect on human physiology. Their sustained experimentation and research, starting in the late 1980s, and continuing to this day, has provided valuable evidence about how the Earth profoundly affects and improves the workings of the body.

To Jeff Spencer, D.C., a master at improving the performance of elite athletes and making them more resistant to the ravages of fierce competition. His unique experience at the highest and most challenging level of sports dramatically demonstrates that optimum performance, whether on the playing field or in everyday activities, benefits immensely from Earthing. Jeff was named Sports Chiropractor of the Year in 2004 by the International Chiropractic Association.

To Jim Healy, a preeminent global figure in cutting-edge medical monitoring technology, for greatly appreciated guidance and support.

To Elizabeth Hughes, for sharing her very personal history of how Earthing relieved her from years of baffling ailments so common to many women, but especially for her tireless and dedicated assistance, in small ways and large, on behalf of Earthing research.

To Dick Brown, Ph.D., the internationally renowned exercise physiologist and trainer of elite athletes, whose research on delayed-onset muscle soreness documented the unique power of Earthing to reduce recovery time from injury.

To San Diego health researcher Dale Teplitz for being such an integral cog in Earthing's scientific detective work in the early days and beyond, and for sharing her dramatic story of healing, as well as her insights after leading many hundreds of individuals to the benefits of Earthing.

To old friends Corky and Kathleen Downing for support and enthusiasm over the years, and for helping show truckers and motorists how to bypass common driving tension and aches with a simple grounded seat pad.

To Sheila Curtiss and Bob Malone, for their stories and for being such staunch Earthing advocates for so long.

To Maurice Ghaly, M.D., who took the time to consider the concept of Earthing and then report about its benefits in the medical literature.

To Russell Whitten, D.C., the first physician to apply Earthing in clinical practice and witness its great healing potential.

To Gabriel Cousens, M.D., Richard Delany, M.D., Martin Gallagher, M.D., D.C., David Gersten, M.D., Louis Gordon, B.Ac.,Tracy Latz, M.D., Wendy Menigoz, D.N., Tina Michaud-Gray, R.N, L.M.T, Chuck Munier, D.M.D., David Richards, M.B.B.S., Amanda Ward, N.D., and R. J. Wilson, M.B. Ch.B., FRACGP, for sharing their perspective in how Earthing adds to their ability to treat and heal patients.

To San Diego veterinarian Steve Blake, D.V.M., who long ago discovered the importance of direct contact with the Earth for indoor animals.

To Bryan Moses, for introducing Earthing to the unique circle of people he helps to keep healthy.

To Bruce Beckert, a luminary in the fabric business, who has always been available, with patience, enthusiasm, and brilliance, to continually help refine the design and conductivity of Earthing devices.

To Nick and Carmen Warren, for sustained support and helping so much to locate and obtain the bits and pieces needed for ever-changing Earthing devices.

To John Gray, Ph.D., bestselling author of *Men Are from Mars, Women Are from Venus,* and healthy lifestyle guru David Wolfe, for sharing their Earthing stories.

To Alix Mayer, Brianna Anderson-Gregg, Shane Austin, Jim Bagnola, Karen Ball, Ted Barnett, Simon Beck, Arvord Belden, Jim Bellacera, Olivia Biera, Gaby Buiskool, Clover Calvet, Armida Champagne, Lynne Corwin, Graeme Dalton, Sara Damskier, Melissa Dawahare, N.D., Lynn Deen, Paul Dunn, Shirley Evans, Henry Falcon, Cynthia and Dennis Fertal, Steve Garner, Randy Gillett, Brad Graham, Janis Horton, Scott Hyatt, Daryl James Jr., Ken Jones, Ashley Kane, Minja Karvinen, H. M. Kearney, Doree Lane, Gail LePine, Dean Levin, John Steve Lopez, Mary Mason, Katie McGuinness, Eileen McKusick, Roberta Mikkelsen, Edie Miller, Mike Miller, Jodie Mitchell, Anita Moran, Stephanie and Chike Okeafor, David Olerud, Roland Perez, Ron Petruccione, Tino Phuthego, Terry Pocklington, Anita Pointer, Jill Queen, Howell Runion, Michael Sandler, Wendy Saunders, Tommy Saville, Jim Schmedding, Don Scott, Rocky Seward, Beverley Shoemaker, Step Sinatra, Donna Tisdale, Katherine Van Hatten, Fabio Luiz Vieira, M.D., Cindy Walsh, Tim Walter, Sandra Wong, and Donna Zerger for sharing their Earthing stories.

To Dan and Tim Hall, Dan Chittock, Steve Kroschel, Jim Lind, Linda

McNair, Anand Wells, Claus Henriksen, Erja Pauninsalo, Jan van Stiphout, and Frédéric Gana, for connecting us to "Earthers" throughout the world.

To William Amalu, for validating the power of Earthing with thermography.

To Christy Westen, D.C., for organizing a survey of Earthing's rapid effects on women's vitality.

To Mel Cheskin, M.B.S., C.Ped., for sharing his expertise on feet, footwear, and grounding.

To Geral Blanchard, L.P.C., a Des Moines psychotherapist, anthropologist, and author of *Ancient Ways: Indigenous Healing Innovations for the 21st Century*, for sharing his insights on the barefoot Hadzabe people of Tanzania.

To E. W. Kellogg, III, Ph.D., for offering concrete suggestions at the epigenetic and molecular levels.

To Faizullah Kakar, Ph.D., Minister for Advising the President of Afghanistan on Health and Education Affairs and National Focal Point for Eradicating Polio, for sharing his enthusiasm of Earthing and history of his country's barefoot warriors.

To author Jed Diamond, Ph.D., an expert on male stress, for introducing his readers to one of the most natural, stress-busting things they can do—ground themselves.

To Marika Sboros, health news editor at South Africa's *Business Day* newspaper, for sharing her insights on what may be the world's biggest medical experiment.

To George Verdon, hale and hardy in his eighties, who has been spending countless barefoot hours in his garden over the last thirty years, for sharing with us his translation of the amazing insights of French agronomist Matteo Tavera.

To Mark Lindsay, for opening research doors.

To John Sullivan, for continuing support and videography.

To Jennifer Morris, for providing much appreciated administrative assistance.

To CJ Puotinen, a veteran pet writer and author, who has experienced how Earthing helps both four- and two-legged creatures.

To Norm Goldfind, a master of the publishing arts, for seeing the potential in our book.

To Cheryl Hirsch, for absolutely superb editing, and to Gary Rosenberg and Terry Wiscovitch, for a beauty of a book.

To Mark Hinds and staff naturopath Anna Walden at the HealthWalk Integrative Wellness Center in Carlsbad, California, for providing zeta potential expertise and sophisticated instrumentation, plus much appreciated patience and assistance.

And to so many others, especially early on, who were willing to try the strange idea of a guy from the cable TV industry with no scientific or medical background who claimed that, by standing barefoot on the Earth or sleeping on a bed pad or sheet connected to the Earth with a wire, you could actually sleep better, feel better, have less pain, and reduce multiple symptoms of illness.

Index

About the Authors

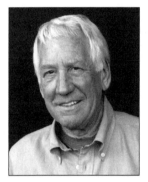

Clinton Ober started as a cable TV salesman in Billings, Montana, and rose to become a leader in the industry. In the early 1970s, he formed Telecrafter Corporation and built it into the largest provider of cable marketing and installation services in the United States. In the 1980s, he turned his attention to the fledgling computer industry. He partnered with McGraw-Hill to acquire live-feed distribution rights for computer use from news services around the world. Following a near fatal disease in 1993, he embarked on a personal journey looking for a higher purpose in life. During his travels, he discovered Earthing and has been resolutely focused ever since to promote the scientific exploration and practical applications for the concept.

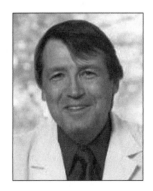

Stephen T. Sinatra, M.D., F.A.C.C. (Fellow of American College of Cardiology), F.A.C.N. (Fellow of American College of Nutrition) is a board-certified cardiologist and certified bioenergetic psychotherapist with forty years of clinical experience treating, preventing, and reversing heart disease. He is also certified in antiaging medicine and nutrition. In his practice, Dr. Sinatra's focus has been integrating conventional medical treatments for heart disease with complementary nutritional, anti-aging, and psychological therapies to counteract the inflammation and plaque processes that cause heart attacks and strokes. He is a fellow of the American College of Cardiology, an assistant clinical professor of medicine at the University of Connecticut School of Medicine, and a former chief of cardiology and medical education at Manchester (Connecticut) Memorial Hospital. A prolific author, Dr. Sinatra has written numerous books, including *The Great Cholesterol Myth* (Fair Winds Press, 2012), *The Sinatra Solution: Metabolic Cardiology* (Basic Health Publications, 3rd ed., 2011), *Reverse Heart Disease Now* (Wiley, 2008), *Lower Your Blood Pressure in Eight Weeks* (Ballantine Books, 2003), *Heart Sense for Women* (LifeLine Press, 2000), and *Heartbreak & Heart Disease* (Keats, 1999). He is also the host of the Internet's leading integrative cardiology website, www.heartmdinstitute.com.

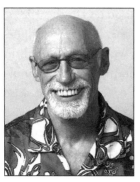

Martin Zucker has written extensively on natural healing, fitness, and alternative medicine for more than thirty-five years. He has co-authored or ghostwritten more than a dozen books. Among his latest books are *Move Yourself* and *Reverse Heart Disease Now* (both from John Wiley & Sons, 2008), *Natural Hormone Balance for Women* (Pocket Books, 2002), *The Miracle of MSM* (Berkley Trade, 1999), *Preventing Arthritis* (Berkley Trade, 2002), *The Veterinarians' Guide to Natural Remedies for Dogs/Cats* (Three Rivers Press, 2000), and *The Miracle of MSM* (Berkley Trade, 1999). Zucker has written hundreds of magazine articles on a wide variety of health topics and contributed to *Smithsonian, Readers Digest, Los Angeles Times, Cook's Magazine, Vegetarian Times, Muscle & Fitness, Men's Fitness,* and *The National Enquirer.* He is a former Associated Press foreign correspondent who worked in Europe and the Middle East.